Oklahoma Notes

Basic Sciences Review for Medical Licensure
Developed at
The University of Oklahoma College of Medicine

Suitable Reviews for:
United States Medical Licensing Examination
(USMLE), Step 1

Oklahoma Notes

Pharmacology

Fourth Edition

Edited by
Joanne I. Moore

With Contributions by
H. Dix Christensen   K. Roger Hornbrook
Sharon L. Jones   Michael C. Koss
Joanne I. Moore   Eugene Patterson
Lester A. Reinke   Lora E. Rikans

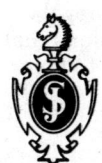

Springer-Verlag
New York Berlin Heidelberg London Paris
Tokyo Hong Kong Barcelona Budapest

Joanne I. Moore, Ph.D.
Department of Pharmacology
College of Medicine
Health Sciences Center
University of Oklahoma
Oklahoma City, OK 73190
USA

Library of Congress Cataloging-in-Publication Data
Pharmacology / edited by Joanne I. Moore ; with contributions by H.
  Dix Christensen . . . [et al.]. — 4th ed.
      p.   cm. — (Oklahoma notes)
    Includes bibliographical references.
    ISBN 0-387-94394-3
      1. Pharmacology—Examinations, questions, etc.   2. Pharmacology—
  Outlines, syllabi, etc.   I. Moore, Joanne I.   II. Christensen, H.
  Dix.   III. Series.
      [DNLM: 1. Pharmacology—examinations questions.   2. Pharmacology—
  outlines.   QV 18 P53605 1995]
  RM301.13.P473   1995
  615′.1—dc20
  DNLM/DLC
  for Library of Congress   94-43678

Printed on acid-free paper.

Production managed by Jim Harbison; manufacturing supervised by Jacqui Ashri.
Camera-ready copy prepared by the editor.
Printed and bound by Edwards Brothers, Inc., Ann Arbor, MI.
Printed in the United States of America.

9 8 7 6 5 4 3 2 1

ISBN 0-387-94394-3 Springer-Verlag New York Berlin Heidelberg

Preface to the
Oklahoma Notes

In 1973, the University of Oklahoma College of Medicine instituted a requirement for passage of the Part 1 National Boards for promotion to the third year. To assist students in preparation for this examination, a two-week review of the basic sciences was added to the curriculum in 1975. Ten review texts were written by the faculty: four in anatomical sciences and one each in the other six basic sciences. Self-instructional quizzes were also developed by each discipline and administered during the review period.

The first year the course was instituted the Total Score performance on National Boards Part I increased 60 points, with the relative standing of the school changing from 56th to 9th in the nation. The performance of the class since then has remained near the national candidate mean. This improvement in our own students' performance has been documented (Hyde et al: Performance on NBME Part I examination in relation to policies regarding use of test. J. Med. Educ. 60: 439–443, 1985).

A questionnaire was administered to one of the classes after they had completed the Boards; 82% rated the review books as the most beneficial part of the course. These texts were subsequently rewritten and made available for use by all students of medicine who were preparing for comprehensive examinations in the Basic Medical Sciences. Since their introduction in 1987, over 300,000 copies have been sold. Obviously these texts have proven to be of value. The main reason is that they present a *concise overview* of each discipline, emphasizing the content and concepts most appropriate to the task at hand, i.e., passage of a comprehensive examination over the Basic Medical Sciences.

The recent changes in the licensure examination that have been made to create a Step 1/Step 2/Step 3 process have necessitiated a complete revision of the Oklahoma Notes. This task was begun in the summer of 1991 and has been on-going over the past 3 years. The book you are now holding is a product of that revision. Besides bringing each book up to date, the authors have made every effort to make the tests and review questions conform to the new format of the National Board of Medical Examiners. Thus we have added numerous clinical vignettes and extended match questions. A major revision in the review of the Anatomical Sciences has also been introduced. We have distilled the previous editions' content to the details the authors believe to be of greatest importance and have combined the four texts into a single volume. In addition a book over neurosciences has been added to reflect the emphasis this interdisciplinary field is now receiving.

I hope you will find these review books valuable in your preparation for the licensure exams. Good Luck!

Richard M. Hyde, Ph.D.
Executive Editor

Preface

More than twenty years ago, the faculty members of the Department of Pharmacology at the University of Oklahoma College of Medicine developed a review book of medical pharmacology in response to requests from our second year medical students who were preparing to sit for the Part I examination of the National Board of Medical Examiners. The students expressed a need for an organized approach to cope with the volume of basic science curricular material presented during the first two years. *Therefore, this book was not developed as a comprehensive text, but rather was designed specifically to provide students with a synopsis of the basic core of information we deemed essential for their review.*

This book represents a major revision of our review of medical pharmacology. It has been updated and expanded, provides current information on major new drugs and information on older drug groups that typically have been covered on previous licensure examinations. Included are a number of new questions for self-examination. The faculty have endeavored to retain a reasonably concise, relevant, and readable review book that will provide the students with a thorough review of pharmacology. Students are advised to refer to comprehensive textbooks, as needed, to fill in any gaps in their knowledge which may be disclosed by the self-examinations.

We wish to acknowledge the help of several contributors to the original and the preceding revisions of the review book. These include former members of the faculty, Daniel M. Byrd, III, Ph.D., John M. Carney, Ph.D., Andrew T. Chiu, Ph.D., Charles F. Meier, Jr., Ph.D., and Walter N. Piper, Ph.D., as well as a Visiting Professor from The University of Michigan, Henry H. Swain, M.D.

We wish to offer our special thanks to a former staff member, Annie M. Harjo, for her skills with the word processor and for remaining calm and unflappable during our efforts in assembling the original book and previous editions. Holly Whiteside deserves our kudos for her contributions to the present edition of *Oklahoma Notes: Pharmacology.*

Joanne I. Moore, Ph.D.
Oklahoma City

Contents

8   The Endocrine System
(K. R. Hornbrook, L. A. Reinke and L. E. Rikans)

9   Anti-Infective Agents
(L. A. Reinke and L. E. Rikans)

10   Cancer Chemotherapy and Immunosuppressive Agents
(L. E. Rikans)

11   Chemotherapy of Parasitic Diseases
(J. I. Moore)

12   Gastrointestinal Drugs
(J. I. Moore)

CHAPTER 1: <u>GENERAL PRINCIPLES</u>

I. **MECHANISMS OF DRUG ACTION**

    A. KNOWN PHYSICAL OR CHEMICAL INTERACTIONS

        1. Osmotic cathartics and osmotic diuretics
        2. Antacids

    B. UNKNOWN MECHANISM RELATED TO A PHYSICAL PROPERTY OF THE AGENT: THE OIL: H_2O SOLUBILITY COEFFICIENT WHICH DETERMINES CELLULAR CONCENTRATION.

        1. CNS depression caused by volatile general anesthetic agents and volatile solvents

    C. MOLECULAR SITE OF INTERACTION: CONCEPT OF DRUG RECEPTORS

        1. Drugs usually are not accumulated at site of action.
        2. Drugs usually do not directly affect known enzymatic pathways or structural elements within cells, although important exceptions occur in chemotherapy and some metabolic effects of drugs.
        3. Most drug effects are produced by interaction with a cellular binding site located in the plasma membrane or intracellularly. By the translation of binding into an observable effect the site is a drug receptor, by definition. The chemical structure of the receptor for some neurotransmitters and hormones has been determined. All are proteins either single chains or various numbers of subunits.
            a. binding not translated into an effect is a storage site (<u>i.e.</u>, plasma protein).
            b. binding at both receptors and storage sites is usually reversible and occurs by low energy forces. A few examples of drug action associated with covalent binding are known (i.e., organophosphorus cholinesterase inhibitors and some chemotherapeutic agents).
                1. covalent binding of drugs or their reactive metabolites to cellular constituents may result in toxicity (<u>i.e.</u>, cellular necrosis, allergic potential, carcinogenesis).
            c. the receptor normally interacts with endogenous substances (<u>i.e.</u>, neuro-transmitters, hormones, autacoids, peptides, etc.); thus the binding of drugs to the receptor requires structural specificity and often stereospecificity.
            d. selective effect of a drug for an organ system is related to the presence of a specific receptor; the type of response is related to the organ's normal function.

D. CHARACTERIZATION OF RECEPTORS

1. Mobile and fixed intracellular receptors - steroid and thyroid hormones; retinoids
    a. complex formed in cytoplasm and derivative goes to nucleus (steroids) or receptor present in nucleus (thyroxin).
    b. production of effect related to synthesis of a specific m-RNA and of new protein molecules.
    c. transduction involves interaction of receptor derivative with DNA; amplification involves the number of new protein molecules synthesized.
2. Fixed cell membrane receptors - catecholamines, acetylcholine and other endogenous substances, or drugs.
    a. interaction generally occurs on or in plasma membrane.
    b. the receptor may modify the activity of transmembrane enzymes, ion channels, guanine nucleotide binding proteins or other processes. These are the transduction processes; amplification is related to increased enzymatic activity or ionic flux.
       1. transmembrane enzymes
           a. protein tyrosine kinases- receptors for trophic factors such as insulin.
              1. transduction and amplification multifaceted. Some occurs through autophosphorylation of receptor and phosphorylation or dephosphorylation of cytosolic proteins. Mechanisms not involving phosphorylation may relate to changes in insulin receptor configuration.
           b. other enzyme-linked transmembrane receptors include: guanylyl cyclase (atrial naturetic factor), tyrosine phosphatases and serine kinases.
       2. ion channels - receptors for some neurotransmitters.
           a. endogenous compounds change the flow of sodium, potassium, chloride and other ions through specialized membrane pores. Voltage-dependent calcium channels are site of action of calcium channel blockers. Many toxins act on these and other channels.
           b. the most studied is the nicotinic receptor for acetylcholine which changes sodium flux. Multisubunit protein; other ion channels also have several subunits and some homology.
           c. drugs mimic or block the action of the endogenous ligands or hinder ion flow through pore.
           d. transduction and amplification related to the enzymatic reactions affected by the ions intracellularly and the number of ions gated.
       3. plasma membrane receptors and the formation of second messengers.
           a. guanine nucleotide binding proteins (G-proteins) are transducers of information between ligand-receptor binding and the formation of several intracellular second messengers. Many G-proteins have been identified, most without a clear function.
              1. stimulation (G_s) or inhibition (G_i) of adenylate cyclase (cyclic-AMP formation).

       2. stimulation of phospholipase C (formation of inositol triphosphate [IP$_3$] and diacylglycerol; and release of intracellular calcium ion).

       3. some ion channels; important effects on potassium channels.

     b. other mechanisms of transduction

       1. formation of cyclic-GMP

       2. formation of prostaglandins and related compounds (phospholipase A$_2$)

       3. formation of free radicals

       4. formation of low molecular weight peptides or glycosyl-phosphatidylinositol from glycophospholipid anchor of proteins in membranes

       5. formation of calcium-calmodulin complexes

       6. formation of nitric oxide from arginine. Increases cyclic-GMP and NO may have direct actions particularly in bacterial killing

     c. protein phosphorylation - function may be increased or decreased

       1. cyclic-AMP dependent protein kinase

       2. cyclic-GMP dependent protein kinase

       3. protein kinase C - regulated by calcium and diacyglycerol; stimulated by phorbol esters

    4. calcium-calmodulin dependent protein kinase; calmodulin also may affect some enzymes (i.e. phosphodiesterase) by a mechanism independent of phosphorylation

    5. phosphoprotein phosphatases - serine phosphate specific, some inhibited by okadaic acid; tyrosine phosphate specific, primarily membrane bound; little known about regulation

3. Desensitization: tolerance; tachyphylaxis-applied primarily to pharmacotherapeutic agents

    a. slow regeneration from inactive receptor form.

    b. formation of endogenous inhibitor.

    c. negative co-operativity of drug-receptor binding.

    d. phosphorylation of receptor; uncoupling of receptor and G-proteins

    e. agonist-mediated decrease in receptor number: down- regulation, internalization.

    f. depletion of "second messenger" or endogenously released factor.

    g. desensitization does not occur with antagonists.

    h. cellular tolerance associated with some CNS drugs probably is not related to changes in drug-receptor interactions but to modifications in the transduction process; physical dependence generally occurs also.

4. Resistance-applied primarily to chemotherapeutic agents

    a. defined as an acquired and inheritable decrease in response to treatment.

    b. general mechanisms

       1. mutation-change in existing protein structure or function.

       2. gene transfer-bacterium to bacterium; R-plasmid; acquisition of new protein.

       3. gene amplification-bacteria and cancer cells; increased amount of existing target or transport protein.

4

c. biochemical mechanisms
1. increased metabolism of drug to inactive product - <u>beta</u> - lactamases and others.
2. decreased intracellular drug concentration - porins
3. increased drug efflux - P170 (P-glycoprotein) and others.
4. increased metabolite which antagonizes drug action - PABA.
5. altered amount of target enzyme or receptor.
6. decreased affinity of receptor for drug-dihydrofolate reductase.
7. enhanced repair mechanisms - DNA repair.
8. decreased activity of an enzyme required to express drug effect - autolysins in bacterial cell walls.
5. Pathologic states of receptor function
a. immunological decrease in number; myasthenia gravis, asthma.
b. agonist-mediated decrease in number; diabetes mellitus, asthma.
c. loss of coupling factor (G-protein) between membrane and cytosol; pseudohypoparathyroidism.
d. excesses and deficiencies in thyroid and/or adrenocortical hormone may change receptor number or magnitude of post-receptor events.

E. CLASSIFICATION OF DRUGS INTERACTING WITH RECEPTORS

1. Agonists - bind to a receptor and produce a response. Generally have structural similarity to endogenous compounds. The magnitude of response for any given concentration of drug is a function of a "stimulus" to the receptors. This in turn is determined by efficacy (a drug property); and by the affinity of the drug for receptors and by the total number of receptors (both tissue properties). "Intrinsic efficacy" is the amount of "stimulus" an agonist applies to each receptor. "Relative efficacy" relates to the percentage of total receptors which must be occupied to produce a given response. These terms are used to compare agonists acting at the same receptor.
a. "full" or "strong" agonists are drugs of "high" intrinsic efficacy which do not have to occupy all of the receptors to produce a maximal response. Thus, there are "spare" receptors for these compounds. Relative efficacy may vary within a series of agonists; that is, two agonists will occupy different numbers of receptors for any given response even though both are full agonists.
b. "partial" or "weak" agonists are drugs with "low" intrinsic efficacy which have to occupy all available receptors to produce their maximal response. No "spare" receptors exist for partial agonists. Tissue factors (receptor number and/or receptor coupling to transduction mechanisms) may cause markedly different relative responses for the same partial agonist when applied to different tissues. Partial agonists antagonize full agonists at sufficient concentration (mixed agonist-antagonist). Final response of the combination is that of the partial agonist alone, which may approach zero. Partial agonists may have greater affinity for receptors than full agonists of the same series.

    c. inverse agonists are drugs which cause an effect opposite to more established agonists and this action is inhibited by specific antagonists for the receptor. This action implies tonic activity in the tissue.

2. Antagonists - drugs that act by inhibiting the action of known endogenous mediators. These are agents with high affinity for the receptor but produce no effect because they lack efficacy. Some drugs classified as agonists may in fact block unknown endogenous substances. Best known antagonists are those which interact with the autonomic nervous system. Structural similarity to agonists is variable and may not be apparent because antagonism results in part from hydrophobic interactions with the receptor. Classification of antagonists is discussed below.

F. QUANTIFICATION OF DRUG-RECEPTOR INTERACTIONS

1. Responses to drugs may be graded (response proportional to dose) or quantal (all or none; dosage required to produce a prestated response, i.e., death or 50 mm increase in blood pressure). Quantal responses may be plotted as a normal distribution histogram or as a cumulative distribution curve. This latter dose-response curve resembles in shape dose-response curves for graded responses. Conceptually, for drugs producing graded responses, the kinetics are the same as enzyme kinetics because the mass action principle is involved in each case.

2. For either graded or quantal responses, dose-response curves are usually presented as $\log_{10}$ dose on the X-axis and the arithmetic response on the Y-axis. The resulting curve is sigmoidal and linear through the middle 66% of the curve. The entire curve can be made linear by converting the percent responses values to probits. Whole probit numbers are 1-3 standard deviations either side of the average response. This plot has most usefulness in drug safety studies (see below) as the responses to very high or very low doses are on the linear portion of the curve.

3. Most accurate point for either type of curve is the dose producing a 50% response (ED_{50}) and comparisons between drugs are usually made at this point. With full agonists, observed ED_{50} may be considerably less than dissociation constant measured by binding of radioactive ligands due to "spare" receptors; i.e., full response is observed with less than 100% occupation.

4. Potency is related to the affinity of the drug for the receptor. Figure 1 (page 7) shows dose-response curves for two agonists, plotted logarithmically. Drug A is more potent than Drug B; it has greater affinity for the receptor and a lower dissociation constant. Potency can be estimated also from the dosage of two drugs required to cause a prestated effect. A more potent drug is not necessarily a better drug. Often potency and toxicity go together because the toxic response is an extension of the therapeutic effect. Changes in receptor number, i.e., an increase as occurs with denervation, will increase the maximal response but not the affinity for the agonist. Changes in response magnitude are not changes in potency.

5. Antagonists can bind to a receptor site or a site near the receptor and thus limit its interaction with agonist.
   a. competitive antagonists shift the dose-response curve for full agonists to the right but do not decrease the maximal response obtainable. In figure 2 (left panel), curve S is the response to agonist R in the presence of a given dose of competitive antagonist. Higher doses of antagonist would cause progressive shifts to the right but no decrease in maximal response (curves T and U). For partial agonists, as all receptors must be occupied for a maximal response, competitive antagonists will decrease the maximal response at sufficient dose (right panel, figure 2; R' - partial agonist alone, S' - partial agonist in presence of competitive antagonist). The amount of depression depends on the rate of dissociation of the antagonist, greater depression as rate slows.
   b. non-competitive antagonists act at a site near the receptor to alter its configuration. Competitive-irreversible antagonists combine covalently with the receptor at the binding site for agonist. For either type of antagonist, the net result is a decrease in apparent receptor numbers. Thus, these antagonists would produce dose-response curves of similar shape. For full agonists, increasing doses of either type of antagonist would shift the curve to the right with no decrease in maximal response until all "spare" receptors are gone and then a decrease in maximal response would occur (figure 3, left panel; X is the response to agonist alone, Y is a response with some "spare" receptors not involved, Z is a response after all "spare" receptors are occupied). For partial agonists, as no "spare" receptors are present, increasing doses of antagonist would cause a progressive decrease in maximal response (figure 3, right panel; X' is the response to partial agonist alone, and Y' and Z' are increasing doses of one of these two types of antagonist).
   c. antagonism of a drug effect by another agent can occur at sites other than the receptor through chemical interactions or opposing functional processes.

G. THERAPEUTIC INDEX

1. An initial evaluation of the safety of drugs using lower animals.
2. Ratio of $LD_{50}:ED_{50}$; might also use a toxic effect (TD_{50}) rather than death as the end point.
   a. curves for toxicity and effect must be parallel for an accurate estimation of the therapeutic index.
   b. not all toxic effects observed subsequently in man will be detected by this screening procedure, i.e., allergic reactions.
   c. certain safety factor, $LD_1:ED_{99}$, gives a better estimate of risk as the slopes of the lines (which may not be parallel) are taken into account. Estimate of value made from probit plots of responses.

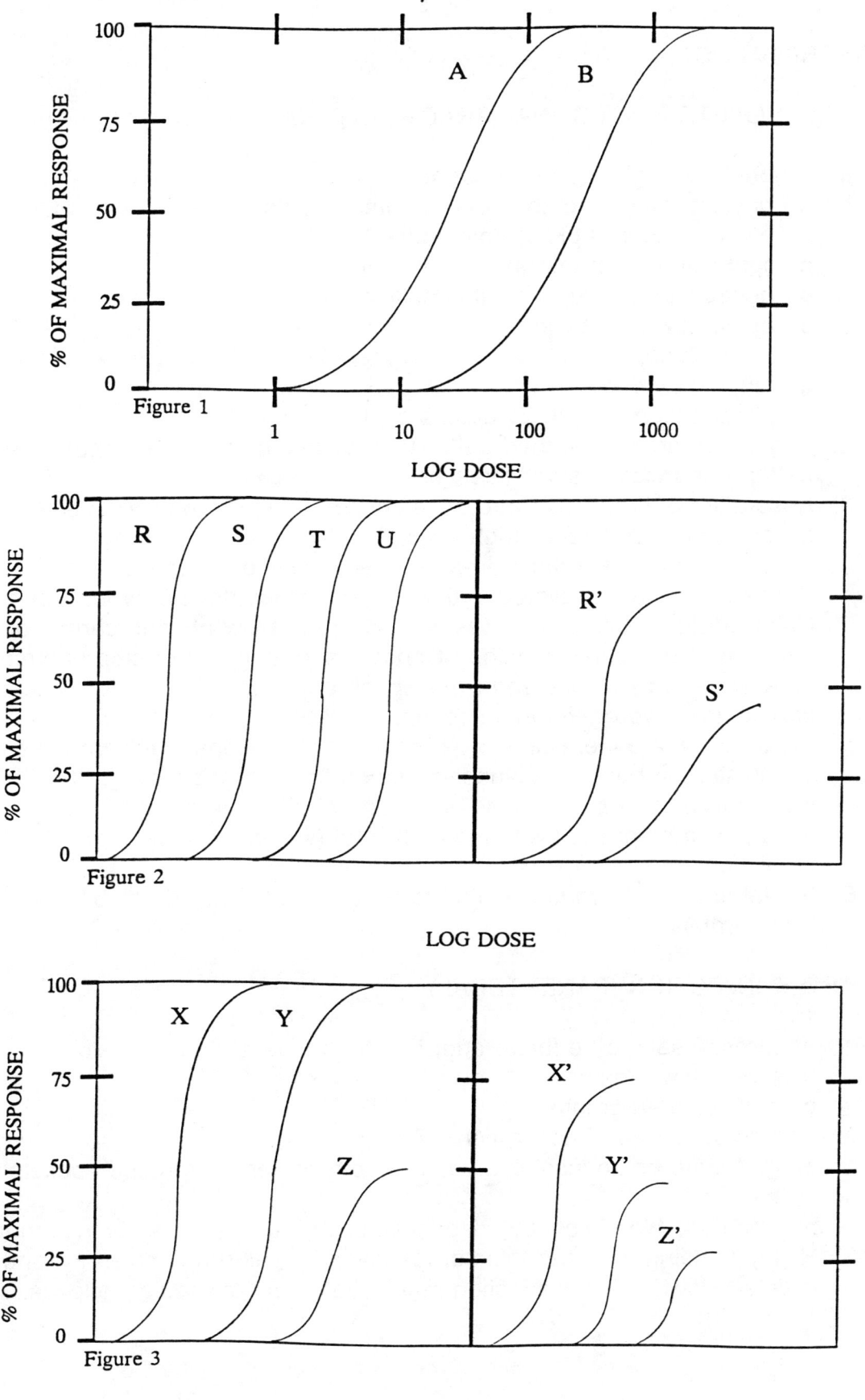

Figure 1

Figure 2

Figure 3

LOG DOSE

II. ABSORPTION OF DRUGS

A. FROM GASTRO-INTESTINAL TRACT (ENTERAL)

1. Amount of drug absorbed depends on:
   a. physical state and solubility in enteral fluids.
   b. pK_a of drug and pH of environment.
   c. lipid solubility of the unionized form.
   d. destruction of drug by gut constituents.
   e. blood flow in gut wall.
   f. transit time.
   g. binding to food.
   h. precipitation of drug by gastric acid.
2. In general, acids absorbed better than bases in stomach; bases absorbed better than acids in small intestine.
3. Absorption of both acids and bases occurs in small intestine because:
   a. pH is not inordinately high - 5.3.
   b. blood flow and surface area of small intestine are large.
4. Bases can be accumulated in the stomach from plasma by ion trapping. Unionized drug diffuses across wall, ionizes at low pH and cannot diffuse back; the converse occurs for acids. Concentrations on either side of membrane can be estimated by Henderson-Hasselbach equation. Energy for accumulation comes from hydrogen ion secretion.
5. Some drugs are ineffective or plasma concentrations highly variable after oral administration because splanchnic blood flow passes through the liver and metabolism occurs (first-pass effect or first-pass metabolism). Rapid liver metabolism by-passed with rectal, buccal (sublingual), or parenteral administration.
6. Rectal and buccal routes limited to drugs with high lipid solubility and little tissue irritation.

B. AFTER INJECTION (PARENTERAL)

1. Absorption said to be faster after i.m. than after s.c.
   a. blood flow greater.
   b. surface area greater.
2. To decrease rate of absorption.
   a. give drug as an insoluble salt or in oil i.m., or compressed pellets implanted s.c.
   b. decrease blood flow by vasoconstriction, generally use epinephrine.
3. Highly irritating or tissue-toxic drugs given i.v.; all drugs given i.v. should be injected slowly. Rapid injection may initiate cardiovascular reflexes.

9

C. OTHER ROUTES

1. Skin - mostly of toxicological importance or for local effect. Scopolamine, nitroglycerin, estrogen and clonidine are exceptions and applied as skin patches.
2. Lungs - gaseous anesthetics and aerosols (local action); latter must have appropriate particle size to reach site of action.

III. DISTRIBUTION OF DRUGS

A. VOLUME OF DISTRIBUTION

1. $V.D. = \dfrac{dose\ (mg)}{plasma\ concentration\ (mg/L)}$

2. This calculation gives V.D. in Liters for a one compartment model.
3. Dividing also by body weight gives value in percent of body weight.
4. Calculated volume may or may not correspond to a body water space.
5. Binding of a drug to a storage site can give a value greater than total body water.
6. V.D. contributes to the rate of elimination of a drug in that the larger the V.D., the slower the rate of elimination.

B. IMPORTANCE OF UNEQUAL DISTRIBUTION

1. Initial distribution to organs which receive a large fraction of cardiac output; subsequent redistribution to less well perfused organs may terminate effect (i.e. thiopental).
2. Blood brain barrier: small capillary pores and glial cells keep compounds with low lipid solubility from interstitial space of brain.
3. Drug storage sites
   a. tissue fat, protein, nucleic acids.
   b. plasma protein.
      1. drugs are bound primarily to albumin, but basic drugs also bind to alpha$_1$-acid glycoprotein.
      2. drug bound to protein is inactive but can serve as storage site and prolong the effect; however, if drug is eliminated by an active process, the effect is shortened because it is carried by the blood to site of elimination.
      3. less binding and more free drug may occur with hypoalbuminemia or uremia.
      4. drug interactions may result because of displacement of a drug bound to plasma protein by a concomitantly administered drug if:
         a. bound drug has a low therapeutic index.
         b. bound drug has a small volume of distribution.
         c. if more than 95% of the drug in plasma is protein bound.

5. increase in free drug concentration after displacement is not sustained because elimination is transiently increased and the original concentration re-established.

IV. EXCRETION OF DRUGS

A. MOST IMPORTANT ROUTE IS THE KIDNEY

1. Drugs filtered at glomerulus can have clearance values between zero and GFR (130 ml/min). The amount passively reabsorbed from the tubules will vary depending on:
   a. pH of urine and pK_a of drug which affect the amount of unionized drug.
   b. lipid solubility of unionized drug.
2. Highly ionized acids and bases are actively secreted by tubular cells and clearance can approach renal plasma flow (600 ml/min).
3. Neonates and elderly have low GFR and low renal blood flow.

B. ENTEROHEPATIC CYCLE

1. Active secretion of a conjugated drug into the bile, i.e., glucuronic acid derivative of a phenol.
2. Unconjugated drug liberated in small intestine after hydrolysis by bacterial enzymes and free drug reabsorbed into plasma.
3. Some drug escapes reabsorption and appears in feces.
4. Antibiotic-induced decreases in intestinal bacterial flora will decrease the hydrolysis of conjugated drugs and may decrease the drug concentration below the therapeutic concentration (sex steroids used for contraception).

C. LUNGS - PRIMARILY ANESTHETIC AGENTS

1. Blood/air partition coefficient.
   a. large value - slow onset and slow excretion (ether). Rate of pulmonary circulation limiting.
   b. small value - rapid onset and rapid excretion (nitrous oxide). Rate of pulmonary ventilation limiting.

D. SKIN: through sweat glands and may result in direct irritation or allergic reactions

V. DETERMINANTS OF PLASMA CONCENTRATION AND DOSAGE SCHEDULES

A. RATES OF ELIMINATION

1. Most drugs disappear from plasma by processes (i.e. metabolism, secretion, filtration) which are concentration dependent (first order or dose-independent kinetics). The higher the concentration, the faster the rate of elimination, up to the amount that the process is saturated.

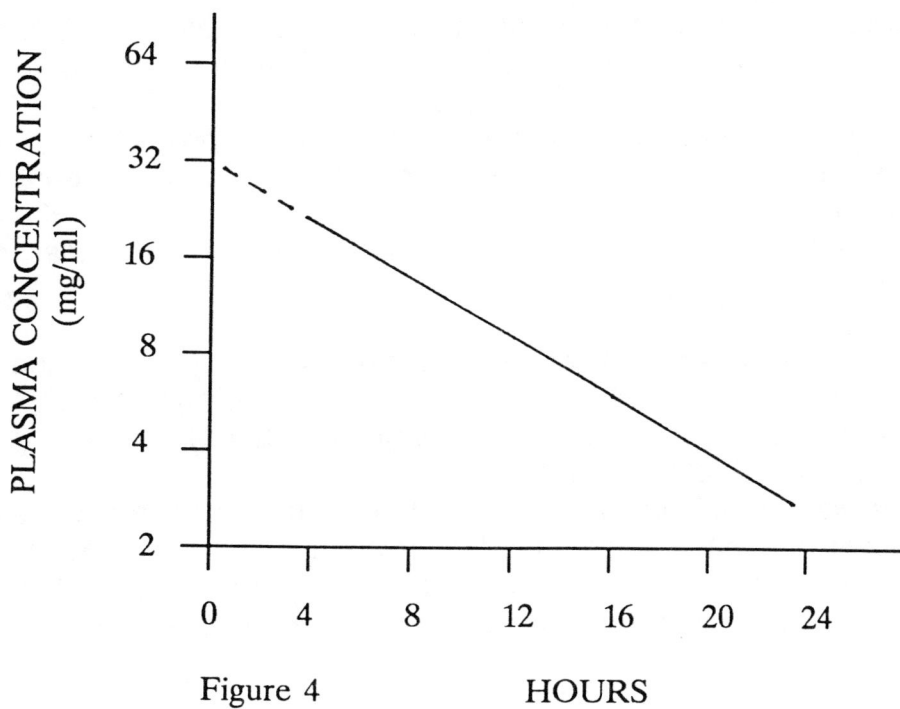

Figure 4   HOURS

a. For drugs which follow first order kinetics, a plot of log plasma concentration against time is a straight line (figure 4). X_o is an extrapolated value and would be the plasma concentration of drug assuming instantaneous distribution.

b. constant percentage of the drug lost per unit time as long as no elimination route is saturated; this value equivalent to the elimination rate constant (k_e).

c. the biologic half-life is constant at all non-saturating plasma concentrations, and is related to k_e:

$$t\frac{1}{2} = \frac{0.69}{k_e}$$

d. k_e and $t\frac{1}{2}$ related to clearance of drug from plasma and volume of distribution:

$$k_e = \frac{clearance\ (ml/min)}{volume\ of\ distribution\ (ml)} = \frac{1}{min} \quad or\ percentage\ of\ drug\ lost\ per\ unit\ time$$

$$or\ t\frac{1}{2} = 0.69 \frac{volume\ of\ distribution\ (ml)}{clearance\ (ml/min)} = min$$

e. these considerations apply only to free drug in plasma and not to that bound to plasma protein.

f. area under the drug elimination curve (AUC) is equal to X_o/k_e and Clearance = $\underline{\text{Dose}}$. By substitution, this formula equivalent to those above.
     AUC

2. Drugs which saturate routes of elimination will disappear from plasma in a non-concentration dependent manner (zero order or dose-dependent kinetics). A slight variant occurs when the drug concentration is near the K_m of the elimination process (Michealis-Menten kinetics). The two variations can be considered together.

    a. plot of log plasma concentration against time may appear linear, particularly at early time periods, but it is illusory. Check graphs closely.

    b. constant amount of drug lost per unit time; there is not an equivalent elimination rate constant.

    c. the biologic half-life is not constant but depends on the concentration; the higher the concentration, the longer the half-life (dose-dependent kinetics).

    d. drugs in this category will demonstrate first order kinetics whenever the drug concentration falls substantially below the K_m of the elimination process.

3. Accumulation of drugs in body

    a. drugs will accumulate until amount administered per unit time is equal to the amount eliminated per unit time (amount in = amount out)

    b. amount in = dose/time
        amount out = plasma concentration (clearance); so:

$$\text{Plasma concentration} = \frac{\text{dose/time}}{\text{clearance}} \text{ or } \frac{\text{infusion rate}}{\text{clearance}}$$

$$= \frac{\text{dose/time}}{\text{volume of distribution } (k_e)}$$

$$= \frac{\text{dose/time}}{\frac{0.69 \text{ (volume of distribution)}}{t\frac{1}{2}}}$$

$$= \frac{1.5 \ (t\frac{1}{2}) \ (\text{dose/time})}{\text{volume of distribution}}$$

    c. this value is the average plasma concentration; the fluctuation around this concentration is equal to the dose administered corrected for volume of distribution. If the volume of distribution is not used, the value is the total drug in the body.

d. the time to reach steady-state concentration is related to t½; 90% of steady state in 3.3 half-lives, 94% in 4 half-lives and 99% in 6-8 half-lives. Drugs with long half-lives (days) may require priming doses to avoid delay in therapeutic effect. An increase in drug dosage does not shorten the time required to reach a steady-state concentration, but will result in a higher plasma concentration.

e. to change concentration, it is generally better to increase the frequency of dosing rather than amount of drug given to avoid toxic effects related to larger excursions around the average concentration.

f. drugs eliminated rapidly (t½ = 4 hr or less) usually given by i.v. infusion or by slowly absorbed preparation.

g. no simple prediction of plasma concentration can be made for drugs eliminated by zero order kinetics. Toxic concentrations can accumulate more quickly and be lost more slowly than drugs which follow first order kinetics.

h. drug dosage in renal disease
   1. applies to drugs excreted primarily (more than 50%) unchanged by kidney and not to those eliminated by other processes.
   2. initial dose same as normal patient.
   3. either dose decreased or dose interval increased in proportion to decrease in renal clearance of creatinine and percentage of drug eliminated unchanged by kidney.

i. no basis for correction of dosage schedules related to hepatic disease.

VI. METABOLISM OF DRUGS

Many drugs are lipophilic, and could remain in the body for prolonged times if they were not transformed into more water-soluble derivatives. Drug metabolism usually decreases the activity of therapeutic agents, but there are important exceptions where active, or toxic, metabolites are formed. Because metabolism plays an important role in determining the duration and intensity of drug action, changes in drug metabolism can become factors in therapy.

The liver is the most important organ for drug metabolism. Some drugs are extensively metabolized in the kidney, lung and intestine, but all tissues appear to catalyze at least some metabolism of drugs.

In the liver, the most important site of metabolism is the endoplasmic reticulum (microsomes) due to the presence of cytochrome P-450. Metabolism of some drugs also occurs in other organelles, such as mitochondria (monoamine oxidase), peroxisomes, and in the cytosol (alcohol dehydrogenase and xanthine oxidase).

A. OXIDATIVE DRUG METABOLISM

1. Cytochrome P-450 - Dependent Oxidations

Most oxidations and reductions (PHASE I reactions) involve the mixed-function oxidase enzymes in the hepatic endoplasmic reticulum. These reactions are catalyzed by the cytochrome P-450 family of hemoproteins, which utilize NADPH and incorporate oxygen into the structure of the drug. Cytochrome P-450 (CYP) enzymes are widely distributed in nature, and more than 300 genes encoding cytochrome P-450 enzymes had been characterized by 1992. Cytochrome P-450 enzymes are divided into families and subfamilies according to their amino acid sequence. For example, CYP 1A2 is from family 1, subfamily A, isozyme 2, and is active in converting many aromatic amines to genotoxic metabolites. Isozymes of the CYP family 2 are most important for drug metabolism, and their levels are also induced by many drugs. Isozymes of the CYP family 3 are also active in drug metabolism, and are induced by many steroids. Isozymes of other CYP families are involved in steroid metabolism and other biosynthetic or catabolic pathways in animals, plants, and microorganisms.

The cytochrome P-450 dependent oxidations include the following:
a. Aromatic hydroxylation
b. Alkyl oxidation
c. Desulfuration
d. Oxidative deamination
e. N-Dealkylation from nitrogen, oxygen and sulfur
f. Sulfoxidation
g. Epoxidation

Metabolites produced by these reactions are usually more water-soluble than the parent compound, and may be excreted as such or processed further by conjugation.

2. Examples of other drug oxidations include:

a. Monoamine oxidase (MAO) in the metabolism of sympathomimetic amines
b. Xanthine oxidase in the catabolism of purines and xanthines
c. Alcohol and aldehyde dehydrogenases

B. REDUCTIVE DRUG METABOLISM

Reductive metabolism generally requires anaerobic conditions, and may be catalyzed by bacteria in the gut or urinary tract. Microsomal enzymes can also reduce drugs under appropriate conditions.

1. Nitro ($-NO_2$) reduction forms corresponding amines (example, chloramphenicol)
2. Organic nitrates are reduced to nitrites
3. Azo ($-N=N-$) bonds are hydrolyzed to form two primary amines

C. DRUG HYDROLYSIS

Drug hydrolysis can occur in plasma, cellular cytosol, and other sites, and can result from chemical or enzymatic reactions. Examples of enzymes are:

1. Esterases (examples; acetylcholine, atropine, procaine)
2. Amidases (examples; procainamide, lidocaine)
3. Peptidases (examples; insulin, vasopressin)

D. CONJUGATION OF DRUGS

Drug conjugations are often referred to as PHASE II reactions, because they often occur after an initial drug oxidation, reduction, or hydrolysis. In most cases, specific transferase enzymes conjugate drugs with cofactors which are normal metabolic intermediates (e.g. acetyl CoA in acetylation; UDP-glucuronic acid in glucuronidation). Because conjugation increases the molecular weight of the drug, these reactions are sometimes classified as SYNTHETIC drug metabolism. The types of drugs conjugations are as follows:

1. Glucuronidation (most significant pathway, many examples). Bilirubin and steroid hormones are important physiological substrates.
2. Sulfation (many examples, including steroid hormones).
3. Glycine and glutamine conjugation of simple aromatic acids (example; salicylates).
4. Glutathione conjugation is an important pathway for removal of reactive metabolites. Mercapturic acids are final excretion products.
5. Acetylation (limited to drugs with primary amino groups such as sulfonamides)
6. Methylation (example; catecholamine O-methyltransferase)

After conjugation, drugs are usually pharmacologically inactive. Glucuronide, sulfate, and glutathione (mercapturic acid) conjugates are highly water soluble, and are readily excreted in the urine.

Conjugation usually increases biliary secretion of drugs. However, enzymes produced by the gut microflora may cleave the glucuronide and sulfate conjugates, and allow the parent drug to be re-absorbed (enterohepatic circulation).

E. FACTORS INFLUENCING DRUG METABOLISM

1. AGE: Fetuses, and newborns generally do not metabolize drugs as well as adults. Drug metabolizing activity usually decreases in old age.
2. SPECIES: Generalization from lower animals to man is often valid, but different metabolites may be formed.
3. GENETICS: Variations in metabolism of succinylcholine, isoniazid and phenytoin can result in toxicity with usual doses of the drugs (see pharmacogenetics section).

4. <u>DISEASE</u>: Various liver diseases can decrease metabolism of many drugs. There are also examples of decreased drug metabolism resulting from cardiac and respiratory diseases, and other extrahepatic conditions.

5. <u>INHIBITION OF DRUG METABOLISM</u>: Competitive inhibition between drug substrate for the microsomal enzymes is readily demonstrated <u>in vitro</u> and can cause exaggerated drug responses <u>in vivo</u>.

   Clinically significant interactions due to decreased metabolism have been reported for anticoagulants, phenytoin and oral hypoglycemic agents, which interact with a diverse group of drugs. These compounds probably get singled out because they are taken chronically in amounts sufficient to saturate drug-metabolizing enzymes and have a low therapeutic index; rather small changes in the plasma concentration may lead to severe, recognizable toxic reactions.

6. <u>INDUCTION OF DRUG METABOLISM</u>: A wide variety of compounds increase the activity of the hepatic microsomal drug metabolizing system. The result is a decrease in pharmacological activity of other concomitantly administered drugs. Barbiturates are classical inducing agents. Induction is usually explained by increases in certain CYP enzymes, but some phase II enzymes may also be increased.

   The magnitude of induction depends on basal level of activity; a two-fold change is common in patients.

7. <u>NUTRITION</u>: Nutritional factors may alter Phase I or Phase II reactions due to the presence of inducing agents in the diet or by affecting the availability of precursors for biosynthesis of cofactors (e.g., carbohydrates for the biosynthesis of UDP-glucuronic acid).

8. <u>HEPATIC CLEARANCE:</u> The liver extracts drugs from the blood with varying degrees of efficiency, and the hepatic blood flow helps to determine whether plasma drug concentrations are altered by changes in activity of the drug metabolizing enzymes. Drugs which are efficiently extracted (high extraction) are affected more by changes in hepatic blood flow than by changes in enzyme activity. Conversely, drugs which are not efficiently extracted (low extraction) are affected more by changes in enzyme activity than by changes in hepatic blood flow.

VII.   PHARMACOGENETICS

Pharmacogenetics is concerned with hereditary abnormal responses to drugs. Pharmacogenetic disorders are inherited in the same way as "inborn errors of metabolism"; however, the condition may not be recognized until the individual is challenged with the drug and exhibits an abnormal response. Investigative approaches to the study of pharmacogenetics include family or twin studies. Some common examples of pharmacogenetic disorders are listed below; many others are known or suspected.

A. ABNORMALLY LOW AMOUNTS OF ENZYME OR DEFECTIVE PROTEIN

1. Succinylcholine Apnea: Caused by an atypical plasma cholinesterase, resulting in prolonged muscle relaxation and apnea after administration of succinylcholine.
2. Acetylation Polymorphism: Rapid and slow acetylators differ by a single autosomal gene. Slow acetylation is a recessive trait. The phenotype determines the rate of N-acetylation of drugs such as isoniazid and sulfonamides. Lupoid reactions from hydralazine and procainamide are more common in slow acetylators.
3. Glucose-6-Phosphate Dehydrogenase Deficiency: The trait is inherited as an X-linked defect, and may result in hemolytic anemia after exposure to primaquine and certain other oxidizing drugs.
4. Abnormalities in Cytochrome P-450: Debrisoquine 4-hydroxylase deficiency was one of the first adverse effects attributed to low levels of a form of cytochrome P-450 (CYP 2D6), which metabolizes many drugs. Similar idiosyncratic drug reactions have been described which can be explained by abnormalities in other CYP enzymes.

B. INCREASED RESISTANCE TO DRUGS

1. Coumarin Resistance: Heritable insensitivity to coumarin anticoagulants; probably related to abnormal proteins which synthesize vitamin K-dependent clotting factors. Affinity is decreased for coumarin, but not for vitamin K.

C. RESPONSES INDIRECTLY RELATED TO DRUG METABOLISM

1. Porphyrias: Induction of the drug-metabolizing enzymes increases heme biosynthesis through increased activity of aminolevulinic acid synthetase. However, slow metabolism of heme precursors in sensitive individuals results in various types of porphyria.

REVIEW QUESTIONS

ONE BEST ANSWER

1. If a drug is excreted into urine as a mercapturic acid conjugate, this indicates that the drug was metabolized by:

   A. Glucuronidation
   B. Sulfate conjugation
   C. Conjugation with methionine
   D. Acetylation
   E. Glutathione conjugation

2. Patients who receive a drug which contains an aromatic amine function (e.g., hydralazine) may require reduced dosage if they:

   A. Are rapid acetylators
   B. Are slow acetylators
   C. Are allergic to barbiturates
   D. Suffer from phenylketonuria
   E. Have a glucose-6-phosphate dehydrogenase deficiency

3. All of the following statements are true of cytochrome P-450 **EXCEPT**:

   A. These enzyme families are found in the endoplasmic reticulum in the liver.
   B. Heme is found at the active site.
   C. Steroid biosynthesis involves cytochrome P-450 enzymes in steroidogenic tissue.
   D. Induction occurs after mutation of genes encoding CYP enzymes.
   E. Most CYP enzymes are capable of metabolizing a wide variety of structurally diverse compounds.

4. Which one of the following is a true statement concerning drugs classified as noncompetitive antagonists?

   A. They increase the maximal response to weak agonists
   B. They generally bind to the receptor through covalent bonds
   C. Dissociation constants of the antagonist for the receptor are 1000 times higher than dissociation constants for the agonists
   D. "Spare" receptors are unaffected by these agents
   E. They bind to the receptor at different sites than the agonist binding site

A new antiarrhythmic agent, "Rhythmstat," is given i.v. to a patient in a dose of 500 mg. The EKG is monitored and blood samples taken for analysis of plasma concentrations. The following concentrations were reported from the laboratory; concentration of free drug in μg/ml.

Time after administration-hours:

0.5	1	2	3	4	5	6	7	8
4.5	4.0	3.4	2.8	2.4	2.0	1.7	1.4	1.3

The EKG tracing showed changes in myocardial conduction for 30 minutes after administration which were indicative of the toxic effect of "Rhythmstat". The patient's PVC's were not apparent in the EKG until 5 hours after the drug was given i.v. The information from the drug company contains no data on the metabolism or renal clearance of the drug. The patient has no pre-existing liver or kidney disease. **Questions 5-8 apply to this data.**

5. The apparent volume of distribution of "Rhythmstat" is about:

   A. 40 liters
   B. 100 liters
   C. 200 liters
   D. 400 liters

ONE BEST ANSWER

6. The patient is sent home with an oral preparation of the drug. You have decided to maintain the average plasma concentration half-way between the toxic and minimal therapeutic plasma concentrations, and to give the drug every eight hours. The dose the patient would take would be within 50 mg of:

   A. 100 mg
   B. 200 mg
   C. 400 mg
   D. 800 mg
   E. 1 gram

7. If the dose of "Rhythmstat" were changed to a bolus dose of 100 mg i.v. every hour, in the steady-state situation the fluctuation in plasma concentration each hour would be about:

   A. 0.1 µg/ml
   B. 1 µg/ml
   C. 10 µg/ml
   D. 100 µg/ml
   E. 1000 µg/ml

8. If the clearance of "Rhythmstat" were only by the kidney, the value calculated would suggest that:

   A. It was filtered and completely reabsorbed
   B. It was filtered and incompletely reabsorbed
   C. It was filtered and not reabsorbed
   D. It was filtered and actively secreted, and thus could be used to measure renal plasma flow
   E. It was filtered and actively secreted but could not be used to measure renal plasma flow

Dose-response curves for the therapeutic effect and the toxic effect of Drug A (left panel) and Drug B (right panel) are given in the figure. The responses are plotted as probits. (9-11)

9. Which one of the following is a true statement concerning the dose-response curves shown above?

   A. The relative efficacy of Drug A is less than that of Drug B
   B. The ED_{50} for Drug A is greater than that for Drug B
   C. The slopes of the dose-response curves would suggest that Drug A and Drug B are acting at the same receptor to produce their therapeutic effect
   D. The slopes of the curves for the therapeutic effect and the toxic effect of Drug B would suggest that the two responses occur by the same mechanisms
   E. Drug A is less potent than Drug B.

10. Which drug has the largest certain safety factor?

    A. Drug A
    B. Drug B
    C. Drug A and Drug B are equally "safe"
    D. Indeterminant

11. Which one of the following statements is the most correct one concerning these dose-response curves?

    A. If the Y axis were the response plotted as a percentage of maximum rather than probits, the resulting curve would be a hyperbola
    B. If the X axis for Drug B were plotted arithmetically rather than as the log dose, the curves for the therapeutic effect and the toxic effect would be parallel
    C. As both drugs appear to produce the same maximal response, this is clear evidence that they are occupying equivalent numbers of receptors when doing so
    D. As the curves for the therapeutic effect and the toxic effect for Drug B are not parallel, this is evidence that Drug B is a weak agonist
    E. When responses to a drug are converted from the percentage of maximum to probits, equal spacing occurs for each standard deviation

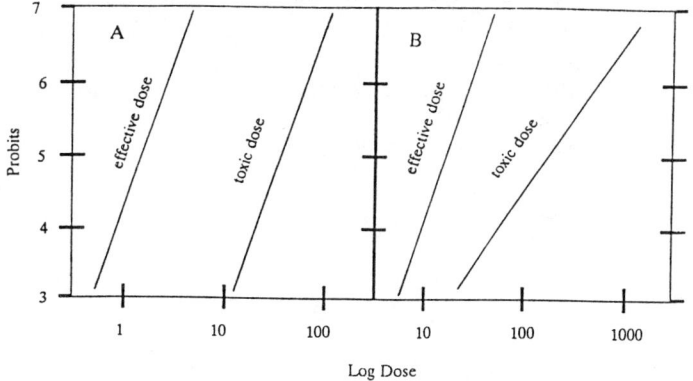

Log Dose

ONE BEST ANSWER

12. Drug X is bound (98%) to plasma protein and has been taken for a sufficient time that the amount in the plasma is at the steady-state. Which one of the following statements would be applicable if another drug (Y), which is bound at the same site on the protein, is given concurrently?

   A. The concentration of free drug X will be increased in plasma as long as Drug Y is given concurrently at sufficient dosage to displace Drug X
   B. As these two drugs bind to the same site on albumin, they must react with the same cellular receptors
   C. The dosage of drug X should be increased because enhanced excretion has resulted in a permanent decrease in its free concentration in the plasma
   D. The total (free + bound) drug concentration of Drug X in the plasma will be decreased at the expense of bound drug
   E. If drugs X and Y were weak acids, the protein to which they are bound would most probably be α_1-acid glycoprotein

Fred Fink complains of heart pain and is admitted to the hospital. He is given an experimental heart numbing drug which can only be given by intravenous administration. The drug has a biological half-life of 3 hours and is given in a dosage of 100 mg/hr. Toxicity is seen when the total body burden is 500 mg. **Questions 13-14 are applicable to this patient.**

13. Which one of the following statements is true concerning Mr. Fink's therapy?

   A. Toxicity would be observed after 9 hours of infusion
   B. Doubling the dose would decrease the time to steady-state
   C. Doubling of the dose would produce a toxic response in 3 hours
   D. The intravenous infusion of 100 mg/hr is without a toxic response
   E. Steady-state never occurs with intravenous administration because constant administration overwhelms the routes for metabolism and excretion

14. Mr. Fink's intravenous therapy continues for 48 hours and then is stopped. Providing Mr. Fink has not stopped also, how long would elapse before the total amount of drug in the body falls to about 56 mg?

   A. 3 hours
   B. 6 hours
   C. 9 hours
   D. 12 hours
   E. Insufficient data to determine

15. Which one of the following statements is applicable to absorption of drugs from the gastrointestinal tract?

   A. Absorption of weak acids occurs only from the stomach and <u>not</u> from the small intestine
   B. All drugs are stable at the low pH of the stomach
   C. Rectal administration is the best way to give irritating drugs
   D. Some drugs are metabolized extensively by the liver and do not reach the general circulation (first pass effect)
   E. Adsorption to food always enhances drug absorption

16. Which one of the following statements is applicable to the binding of drugs at specific sites within the organism?

   A. Drugs which penetrate the blood-brain barrier are excluded from fat stores
   B. Binding of drugs to plasma protein occurs through covalent bonds
   C. Binding to nucleic acids occurs with the same chemical bonds as binding to fat
   D. Hydrophobic bonding is important in determining the affinity of a drug for its receptor
   E. Storage in fat decreases the duration of action of a drug

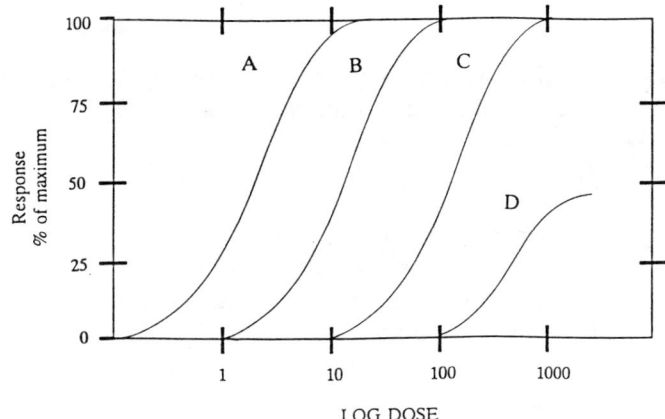

LOG DOSE

17. Which one of the following statements is true concerning the above dose-response curves?

A. Curves A, B, and C represent responses to weak agonists with C being the least potent
B. Curve A represents the responses to a full agonist and curves B and C represent the responses to the agonist in the presence of two concentrations of a competitive antagonist
C. Curves A, B, and C represent 3 drugs which are acting at different receptors as their potencies are different
D. Curve D could be the response to agonist A in the presence of a competitive inhibitor
E. Curve D represents an agonist with a high intrinsic efficacy as the dose needed for a given effect is larger than that of agonists A, B, or C

18. All of the following are true statements about the concept of spare receptors **EXCEPT**:

A. Full agonists have an ED_{50} lower than the estimated dissociation constant of the drug for its receptor
B. Spare receptors do <u>not</u> exist for partial agonists
C. At low doses of a competitive-irreversible antagonist, the response to a full agonist would be shifted to the right with no decrease in maximal response
D. Spare receptors are coupled to second messengers which are different for those for regular receptors
E. Partial agonists act on the same receptors as full agonists

19. A drug is cleared from the plasma into the urine. The clearance value is 130 ml/min and the volume of distribution of the drug is 130 liters. Which one of the following statements would be applicable given this information for the drug?

A. The drug is excreted by both glomerular filtration and active tubular secretion
B. The drug is rapidly metabolized by the hepatic drug metabolizing system
C. The first order rate constant for excretion of the drug (K_e) is .1/ml
D. The drug may be stored in a depot such as adipose tissue
E. This drug would be excluded from the brain

20. All of the following may be associated with phosphorylation of proteins as a primary transduction mechanism **EXCEPT**:

A. Phorbol esters
B. Calmodulin
C. Nicotine
D. Insulin
E. Cyclic-GMP

21. Which one of the following statements is applicable to concept of the "ion-trapping"?

A. Drugs accumulate in fat cells because the high concentration of fatty acids produces a lower pH than that found in plasma
B. Weak bases are more readily excreted by making the urine alkaline
C. Weak acids are well absorbed from the small intestine
D. Weak bases given intravenously will accumulate in the stomach
E. Active secretion of glucuronide conjugates into the bile

ONE BEST ANSWER

22. All of the following are applicable to the concept of the blood-brain barrier **EXCEPT**:

   A. Restricts the entry of hydrophilic compounds into the brain
   B. Has as one component, endothelial cells with pores accessible only by compounds of less than 200 daltons
   C. Is between the plasma space and the interstitial space of the brain
   D. Is penetrated only by organic solvents which are used as general anesthetic agents
   E. Drugs which are well absorbed from the G.I. tract penetrate well into the brain

23. Covalent binding of drugs to body constituents:

   A. Occurs only with competitive antagonists
   B. Occurs with all chemotherapeutic agents
   C. May account for the hematopoietic toxicity of some drugs
   D. Can be readily reversed in isolated tissue preparations by repeated washing of the preparation.
   E. May occur with one stereoisomer of a drug but not the other isomer

24. Which one of the following statements is applicable to drug-receptor interactions?

   A. Intrinsic efficacy is determined primarily by the molecular weight of the drug
   B. Occur only with monomeric transmembrane proteins
   C. Are easily identified with isotope-labelled drugs
   D. Kinetics generally follow the law of mass action
   E. The number of receptors present on the cell has **NO** influence on the response to a drug

25. Formation of inositol triphosphate after a drug-receptor interaction would increase:

   A. Diacylglycerol
   B. Nitric oxide
   C. Calcium release from cellular stores
   D. Cyclic-GMP
   E. Tyrosine kinase activity

26. All of the following statements are applicable to the sublingual route of administration **EXCEPT**:

   A. Plasma concentration decreased by first pass metabolism
   B. Lipid soluble drugs absorbed rapidly
   C. Irritant drugs should not be given by this route
   D. Blood flow through the mucosa is high
   E. Taste of drugs limits the usefulness of this route

27. Nomopus was found by Swampoyle LTD to cause kidney damage and was replaced by ZitsBgone. This latter drug has a biological half-life of 30 minutes. Which one of the following statements is consistent with that observation?

   A. The drug is stored in high concentrations in fat
   B. The rate of disappearance rules out any metabolism of the drug by the liver
   C. The drug may be actively transported into tubular urine
   D. The drug is 25% bound to plasma protein
   E. The drug is eliminated only by glomerular filtration

28. Which one of the following statements is true concerning renal excretion of drugs:

   A. Drug bound to plasma protein is filtered at the glomerulus
   B. All ionized drugs are reabsorbed in the kidney tubule
   C. Urinary pH has **NO** effect on excretion of drugs
   D. Binding of highly ionized drugs to plasma protein will increase their excretion rate
   E. The concentration of drug in the urine is equal to that in the plasma

29. All of the following statements are true concerning the diminished response of an organ following continued application of a drug **EXCEPT**:

   A. Might result from the modification of a receptor so that it does not bind agonists
   B. Is called tachyphylaxis when it occurs rapidly
   C. Might result from the internalization of drug-receptor complexes
   D. Involves only binding to spare receptors
   E. May result from depletion of an endogenous mediator

ONE BEST ANSWER

30. Getoffamycase, an antipsychotic drug, marketed by Parenoid Farmaceuticals, is metabolized in the liver by an enzyme that has a K_m for the drug of 1.0 mg/ml of plasma. This is the only route of its inactivation. The effective plasma concentration is 100 mg/ml. Which one of the following statements would be applicable?

A. If the daily dosage of the drug were doubled, the plasma concentration would increase 1.5 times
B. At the effective plasma concentration, drug loss will follow "dose-dependent" kinetics
C. The same amount of time will elapse while the concentration drops from 100 mg/ml to 50 mg/ml as that for 50 mg/ml to 25 mg/ml
D. The unit for zero order rate constants is 1/time
E. Induction of hepatic drug metabolizing enzymes should increase the plasma concentration

31. All of the following are true statements about the alteration of the drug dosage schedule in a patient with kidney disease **EXCEPT**:

A. Is more easily done than in patients with hepatic disease
B. Generally is done using changes in creatinine clearance
C. Is generally important if the drug is excreted more than 50% unchanged by the kidney
D. The initial dose given to the patient is not changed
E. Is most important for drugs metabolized completely by the liver

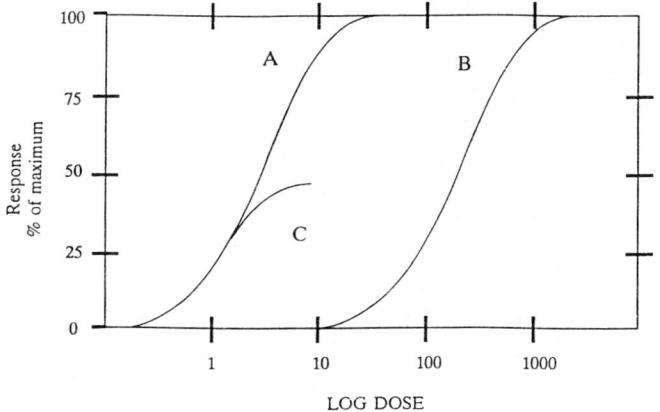

LOG DOSE

32. Drugs A, B and C act on the same receptor. All of the following are true statements concerning these dose-response curves **EXCEPT**:

A. Drug A is a full agonist
B. Drug C is a weak agonist
C. At sufficient concentration, Drug C could antagonize the effects of Drug B
D. Drug A is more potent than Drug C
E. Drug B is a full agonist

33. **Referring to the same graph in question 32**, all of the following statements are applicable to these dose-response curves **EXCEPT**:

A. Curve B might be the response to Drug A in the presence of a competitive inhibitor
B. Curve C might be the response to Drug A in the presence of a noncompetitive inhibitor
C. The intrinsic efficacy of Drug C is less than that of Drug B
D. Mixtures of Drug A and Drug B would give a response like that of Drug C
E. Drugs A and B are full agonists

34. All of the following are true statements concerning the concept of "spare" receptors **EXCEPT**:

A. Maximal effect of partial agonists is obtained only when all receptors are occupied
B. Occupation of all receptors by full agonists will produce a maximal effect
C. The greater the number of receptors, the greater the possibility of an effect at low concentrations of agonists
D. Regular receptors and "spare" receptors have different protein structures
E. "Spare" receptors bind to isotope-labelled agonists with the same affinity as do "regular" receptors

35. Peptide hormones such as insulin, growth hormone and vasopressin usually have a short duration of action because:

A. The wide distribution of non-specific peptidases in the body
B. Rapid urinary excretion
C. Rapid biliary excretion
D. They are excellent substrates for cytochrome P-450

24

ONE BEST ANSWER

36. Enzyme which is important for purine metabolism:

   A. Glutathione S-transferase
   B. Aldehyde oxidase
   C. Xanthine oxidase
   D. Monoamine oxidase
   E. Catechol O-methyltransferase

37. If two drugs which are taken concurrently by a patient are metabolized by the same enzyme system, a clinically significant drug interaction is most likely to occur if:

   A. Both drugs are highly water soluble.
   B. At least one of the drugs is eliminated by "zero order kinetics".
   C. The drugs have a high "therapeutic index".
   D. The metabolites of the drugs have activities close to those of the parent compounds.
   E. One of the drugs has a potentially toxic metabolite.

* * * * * * * * * * * * * *

MATCHING

Choices (may be used more than once):

   A. CYP isozymes
   B. Xanthine oxidase
   C. Monoamine oxidase
   D. Glucuronidase
   E. Catecholamine O-methyltransferase
   F. Alcohol dehydrogenase
   G. Aldehyde dehydrogenase
   H. N-Acetyltransferase
   I. Glucuronyltransferase
   J. Glutathione S-transferase
   K. Plasma esterases

38. Enzyme is often deficient in premature infants, which may cause hyperbilirubinemia

39. Individuals who are homozygous for a form of this enzyme metabolize isoniazid slowly

40. Catalyzes oxidation of norepinephrine

41. Catalyzes conjugation of norepinephrine

42. Metapyrone, which is used to inhibit adrenal glucocorticoid biosynthesis, may have similar effects on hepatic enzymes.

43. Disulfiram is used clinically for treatment of alcoholism because it inhibits this enzyme

44. Hydrolyzes the "prodrug" chloramphenicol sodium succinate to release the active antibacterial drug, chloramphenicol

45. Phenobarbital and many other drugs increase its activity

46-47. Methylxanthines such as caffeine and theobromine are metabolized in two types of oxidative reactions to uric acid derivatives. One of these steps is a demethylation reaction catalyzed by (Question 46), and the second is oxidation to a uric acid derivative which is catalyzed by (Question 47).

48. Forms a tripeptide conjugate with drugs and other chemicals

49. Bacterial enzymes in the gut hydrolyze conjugates after biliary excretion so that the parent drug can be reabsorbed

50. Responsible for the metabolism of ethylene glycol and methanol to toxic products

MATCHING

Abnormal responses to drugs:

A. Malignant hyperthermia with muscular rigidity
B. Exacerbation of porphyria
C. Glucose-6-phosphate dehydrogenase deficiency
D. Increased receptor affinity for menadione

51. Halothane

52. Warfarin

53. Primaquine

54. Phenobarbital

CHAPTER 2: <u>DRUGS ACTING ON THE PERIPHERAL NERVOUS SYSTEM</u>

I. **AUTONOMIC NERVOUS SYSTEM: PARASYMPATHETIC DIVISION (Cholinergic)**

A. FUNCTIONAL

1. Bradycardia <u>via</u> efferent vagus; little or no direct action on contractile force. No parasympathetic tone to blood vessels in general.
2. <u>Eye</u>: main tone to iris; causes miosis upon stimulation - involvement in light reflex - also tone to ciliary body. Blockade leads to mydriasis and cycloplegia; overactivity leads to miosis and spasm of accommodation.
3. Constriction of bronchial tree - of limited significance in man; more so in patients with asthma; increased tone of G.I. tract and urinary bladder; increased G.I. secretions.
4. Parasympathetic stimulation of salivary glands → profuse, watery saliva. Parotid gland innervated only by parasympathetic system.
5. <u>Botulinus toxin</u>: prevents release of ACh; <u>Hemicholinium</u>: prevents reuptake of choline; <u>Black Widow spider venom</u> (latrotoxin): causes excessive release of ACh.
6. Acetyl-CoA + Choline → Acetylcholine; enzyme is choline acetylase. ACh stored in granules; breakdown rapid <u>via</u> specific enzyme called acetylcholinesterase.

B. SYNTHESIS AND TERMINATION OF EFFECT - synthesized by enzyme choline acetyltransferase (choline acetylase) by complexing choline with acetyl coenzyme A to produce acetylcholine. Destruction of acetylcholine is by cholinesterases to produce acetic acid and choline. Acetylcholinesterases located in neuronal membranes and red blood cells; pseudocholinesterase (non-specific or butyrylcholinesterase) more widely distributed.

C. CHOLINE ESTERS

1. <u>Acetylcholine</u>: endogenous neurotransmitter (ACh).
   a. Acts on nicotinic and muscarinic receptors (all parasympathetic end organs; autonomic ganglia; NMJ; adrenal medulla; some sympathetic nerves to skeletal muscle blood vessels and to sweat glands; CNS muscarinic and nicotinic receptors).
   b. The smooth muscle of blood vessels is directly relaxed by small doses of ACh which stimulate non-innervated <u>muscarinic</u> cholinergic receptors; decreases TPR, mean and diastolic BP; the drop in BP will elicit <u>via</u> the baroreceptor mechanism a reflex increase of sympathetic activity. These non-innervated muscarinic receptors are located on vascular endothelial cells and the effect is mediated by release of EDRF (nitric oxide).

c. Direct effects on cardiac <u>muscarinic</u> cholinergic receptors to decrease heart rate (automaticity decreased by decreasing rate of slow diastolic (phase 4) depolarization); speeds conduction of electrical impulses in atrial muscle but slows conduction through the AV node and prolongs refractory period of the AV node; reflex sympathetic activity to speed HR and increase cardiac contractility will oppose direct ACh actions on the heart.

2. <u>Muscarinic receptors</u>: M_1-CNS and sympathetic ganglia; M_2-cardiac; M_3-smooth muscle and glands.

3. <u>Methacholine</u>: ACh with CH_3 substitution; strong muscarinic action; little nicotinic effects; partially refractory to enzyme hydrolysis; following i.v. administration BP falls greatly (blocked by atropine).

4. <u>Carbachol</u>: ACh plus terminal NH_2; strong nicotinic action; lesser muscarinic actions; almost totally refractory to hydrolysis (following atropine, BP increases); also releases ACh; used as miotic.

5. <u>Bethanechol</u>: CH_3 and NH_2 addition to ACh (like both methacholine and carbachol); ester of choice in treatment of urinary retention and to increase G.I. motility. Has mainly muscarinic with some nicotinic actions; refractory to enzyme breakdown.

E. CHOLINOMIMETIC ALKALOIDS

1. <u>Muscarine</u>: classical agent - in part responsible for rapid type of mushroom poisoning; acts strongly on all muscarinic receptors; hypotension; glandular secretions. Physiological effects are reversed by atropine-like drugs.

2. <u>Pilocarpine</u>: muscarinic stimulant; a drug of choice in treatment of glaucoma (contracts ciliary muscle and constricts pupil and thus increases outflow of aqueous humor).

3. <u>Nicotine</u>: isolated from tobacco leaves; nicotinic receptor stimulant; colorless liquid in pure state; activation of NMJ, all ganglia; adrenal medulla; potent CNS excitation; tolerance develops in smokers. Strongly addictive; now used in transcutaneous patches for cessation of smoking.

F. CHOLINERGIC BLOCKING AGENTS

1. <u>Atropine</u>: prototype; orally absorbed and readily enters CNS; selective competitive blockade of muscarinic receptors; also has prominent CNS effects; low doses may slow HR by both direct and CNS actions; larger doses will increase HR and speed conduction of impulses through the AV node; cardiac contractility usually unaffected except at very high dosages which can depress contractility. Low doses will block responses to nerve stimulation or injected cholinergic drugs; decreased G.I. and urinary bladder motility, lack of sweating, and dry mouth; mydriasis and cycloplegia. Little direct effect on B.P. Sometimes used as preanesthetic medication. Very toxic in children; treat with physostigmine; dangerous in glaucoma patients.

2. <u>Scopolamine</u>: like atropine blocks all muscarinic receptors; in adults may cause more sedation than atropine; some use in prevention of motion sickness.

3. Atropine Substitutes: many quaternary ammonium or tertiary amino derivatives synthesized; all closely resemble natural alkaloid; many used in ophthalmology (i.e., homatropine and cyclopentolate) to produce mydriasis and cycloplegia; shorter duration of action. Other drugs commonly used in G.I. and genitourinary conditions (i.e., glycopyrrolate) and for inhalational treatment of asthma (i.e., ipratropium); quaternary amines-less CNS effect.
4. Benztropine: stronger CNS effect; less peripheral action; used in treatment of Parkinson's disease (others discussed in later chapters).

G. ANTICHOLINESTERASE AGENTS - enhance cholinergic function by complexing with enzyme that breaks down ACh (acetylcholinesterase). Signs and symptoms include activation of nicotinic and muscarinic receptors where innervated.

1. Physostigmine: also called eserine, acts only as an anti-AChase. Effects last 4 to 6 hrs.; rarely used clinically for treatment of myasthenia gravis as other drugs are better due to dual action (see below). Rational use would include treatment of atropine poisoning due to entry into CNS, also used to treat glaucoma.
2. Neostigmine: acts like physostigmine but also has direct action on skeletal muscle; one drug of choice for symptomatic treatment of myasthenia gravis; 4-6 hr action; binds to both anionic and ester sites on enzyme. Neostigmine (unlike physostigmine) is excluded from CNS; also common antidote for competitive block of NMJ.
3. Pyridostigmine and Ambenonium: used in treatment of myasthenia gravis especially in patients that have become tolerant to actions of neostigmine. Actions and binding are similar.
4. Edrophonium: short acting; binds strongly only to anionic enzyme site. Useful in diagnosis of myasthenia gravis and "cholinergic crisis".
5. Parathion and Isoflurophate (D.F.P.): "nonreversible" as are very slowly released from enzyme by hydrolysis; bind to ester site on enzyme. Are used primarily as insecticides; some used topically to treat glaucoma. Can be removed from enzyme by oxime reactivators such as 2-PAM (pralidoxime) along with atropine (for muscarinic effects).

II. **AUTONOMIC NERVOUS SYSTEM: GANGLIA**

ACh released at ganglionic synapse.
Adrenal medulla - pharmacologically behaves as a sympathetic ganglion and is stimulated and blocked by agents acting on autonomic ganglia.

A. GANGLIONIC STIMULANTS

1. General Action: stimulates all autonomic ganglia, both sympathetic and parasympathetic. Unique drugs, both stimulants and blockers (dose dependent effects) of autonomic ganglia. Experimental interest - no therapeutic uses - stimulate ganglion cells directly.

2. Agents:
Nicotine (small dose)
DMPP (used for research)
Acetylcholine (large dose)

3. Actions:
Cardiovascular (primarily due to sympathetic stimulation); vasoconstriction, tachycardia, blood pressure elevation, cardiac force and output increased; (secondary-parasympathetic and reflex effects ensue); slowing of heart rate, brief episodes of vagal arrest with escape; cardiac arrhythmias due to imbalance of vagal slowing (mediated via ACh release) vs. increased sympathetic activity (mediated via catecholamine release) to enhance automaticity.

B. GANGLIONIC BLOCKING DRUGS

1. General Action: blockade and inhibition of transmission at both sympathetic and parasympathetic ganglia.
2. Agents:
   a. Hexamethonium (C_6): short acting; N+ group therefore not effective orally.
   b. Chlorisondamine and Mecamylamine: longer acting; orally effective; rarely used today.
   c. Trimethaphan: only agent used today with any frequency; used in surgery to reduce B.P.; ultra short acting = rapid recovery.
   d. d-Tubocurarine: also blocks ganglia at moderate to high concentrations.
   e. Nicotine: large or repeated doses produce depolarization blockade.
3. Effects of ganglionic blockade include:
   a. Decreased blood pressure due to decreased sympathetic tone.
   b. Tachycardia or bradycardia depending on heart rate prior to blockade.
   c. Mydriasis and cycloplegia (dilated pupil and paralysis of accommodation).
   d. Decreased G. I. and urinary tone; dry mouth (xerostomia) and lack of sweating (anhidrosis); dry mouth overcome by muscarinic stimulants such as pilocarpine.
   e. Postural hypotension: reflex adjustments blocked; vasodilation, hypotension, increased peripheral flow, pooling of blood, decreased venous return, and decreased cardiac output.

III. **SOMATIC NERVOUS SYSTEM: NEUROMUSCULAR BLOCKING DRUGS**

A. FUNCTIONAL

1. Depression of neuromuscular function:
Tetrodotoxin - blocks Na^+ conductance; batrachotoxin - increases K^+ conductance; hemicholinium - inhibits choline uptake for synthesis; botulinus toxin - binds to sites on prejunctional membrane and prevents release of ACh; Black Widow Spider venom (latrotoxin) - clumping of vesicles at prejunctional membrane, thus excessive release followed by depression; antibiotics

(neomycin, streptomycin, etc.) depress ACh release; <u>general anesthetics</u> - stabilize membrane, thus inhibit response by ACh; lack of Ca^{++}; snake <u>alpha</u>-toxins bind irreversibly to receptors.

2. Facilitation of neuromuscular function: excess Ca^{++}; catecholamines; anticholinesterase agents (i.e., neostigmine, physostigmine, etc.); K^+ ion.

B. COMPETITIVE AGENTS - compete with acetylcholine for postjunctional receptors at endplate; blockade overcome by anticholinesterase drugs. Quaternary nitrogen prevents entry into CNS and fetus.

1. <u>d-Tubocurarine</u>: produces flaccid paralysis lasting from 10 to 40 minutes; smaller muscles affected first, diaphragm last. Effects potentiated by 1) anesthetics (ether, halothane, and methoxyflurane), and 2) antibiotics (neomycin, streptomycin, kanamycin, etc.). Effects can be reversed by anticholinesterase agents (i.e., neostigmine and edrophonium). Muscarinic blocker usually given prior to reversal to prevent muscarinic effects. Hypotension caused by both release of <u>histamine</u> and ganglionic blockade. No CNS effects. Not analgesic. Myasthenia gravis patients are very sensitive to these agents. Bronchospasm may occur due to histamine release. Mainly metabolized; can be excreted in bile. Also release of heparin.

2. <u>Pancuronium</u>: like above but more potent and much less release of histamine; steroid nucleus. Excreted in urine, thus may create problem in patients with kidney disease. No ganglionic blockade or histamine release.

3. <u>Gallamine</u>: shorter duration than d-tubocurarine; causes selective cardiac vagal blockade. In other respects like pancuronium; no histamine or ganglionic blockade. Contraindicated in cardiac and renal disease.

4. <u>Atracurium</u>: short acting due to spontaneous degradation at physiological pH; about same potency as curare; less histamine release; no CV side effects. Especially suited for patients with impaired hepatic or renal function.

5. <u>Vecuronium</u>: more potent analog of pancuronium; shorter duration due to enhanced metabolism; suitable in patients with renal failure; no significant ganglionic or vagal blockade.

C. DEPOLARIZING AGENTS - produce initial depolarization of endplate (phase I) which over time may develop into a "receptor inactivation" block (phase II). Anticholinesterase agents enhance blockade (during phase I only).

1. <u>Succinylcholine</u>: short acting; used for shorter procedures (5-10 min); also releases histamine. Produces initial fasciculations of muscle and blockade is potentiated by anticholinesterase agents. Broken down by plasma and liver pseudocholinesterase, therefore can cause problems in patients with low levels of this enzyme. Also competes with procaine, etc., for enzyme sites. Can cause an increase in intraocular pressure and cerebrospinal fluid pressure. May trigger "malignant hyperthermia"; treat with dantrolene.

2. <u>Decamethonium (C-10)</u>: similar to succinylcholine, but longer duration of action; older agent, not used clinically.

IV. **AUTONOMIC NERVOUS SYSTEM: SYMPATHETIC DIVISION (Adrenergic)**

A. FUNCTIONAL

1. Only major <u>tone</u> to blood vessels (<u>alpha</u>-adrenoceptors) - neurally elicited decrease of BP due to decrease in sympathetic tone (also mechanism for baroreceptors). Heart rate and contractile force increased due to sympathetic activation - this is a unique action of norepinephrine (NE) acting on the <u>beta</u>$_1$-adrenoceptors.
2. <u>Eye</u>: Dilated iris <u>via</u> sympathetic action on radial muscle.
3. G.I. tract inhibited by sympathetics - both <u>alpha</u> and <u>beta</u>- adrenoceptors. Bronchi dilated primarily by circulating epinephrine acting on <u>beta</u>$_2$ receptor.
4. Sweat glands - part of sympathetic system but ACh is the transmitter at neuroeffector junction (sympathetic-cholinergic).
5. Humoral effects of epinephrine include breakdown of glycogen (glycogenolysis) and free fatty acid release.

B. SYNTHESIS AND TERMINATION - Tyrosine converted by enzyme tyrosine hydroxylase to dopa. Dopa to dopamine and dopamine to norepinephrine <u>via</u> action of dopa decarboxylase and dopamine-<u>beta</u>-hydroxylase (in storage granule) respectively, (first two enzymes are cytoplasmic). Cytoplasmic enzyme in the adrenal medulla (phenylethanolamine-N-methyl- transferase) transfers methyl group to form epinephrine. Norepinephrine and epinephrine have negative feedback action on activity of tyrosine hydroxylase. Termination of action is primarily by reuptake (60-90%) into nerve terminal. Secondary inactivation by MAO (primarily intraneuronal) and COMT (primarily extraneuronal). Both enzymes also in gut wall and liver.

C. CATECHOLAMINES - must have 3,4-OH substitution on benzene ring. COMT acts here (primarily extraneuronal). <u>Alpha</u> carbon (CH_3) substitution protects against MAO which acts primarily within the nerve terminal. Product of breakdown by <u>both</u> MAO and COMT = vanillylmandelic acid (VMA); more correctly called 3-methoxy-4-hydroxy-mandelic acid. This is one of compounds screened for in suspected pheochromocytoma. In CNS, major metabolite is 3-methoxy-4-hydroxy-phenylglycol.

1. <u>Norepinephrine</u>: endogenous neurotransmitter (NE).
   a. Catecholamine released from all sympathetic nerves (except sympathetic-cholinergic system); <u>tyrosine hydroxylase</u> is rate limiting step in synthesis; acts strongly on <u>alpha</u>-but not on <u>beta</u>-adrenoceptors with <u>exception</u> of those in the heart and JG apparatus of kidney (<u>beta</u>$_1$). Direct acting and not effective orally (broken down by MAO and COMT in gut wall and liver).
   b. Stimulates <u>alpha</u>-adrenoceptors (<u>alpha</u>$_1$ and <u>alpha</u>$_2$) in vascular smooth muscle; arterioles in skin and mucosa, splanchnic, renal and coronary

vascular beds directly constricted; TPR, diastolic and systolic BP increase; veins also constricted; increased BP activates baroreceptors to reflexly decrease sympathetic tone and to increase vagal activity.

c. Direct effect on beta$_1$-adrenoceptors of heart to increase heart rate, force and velocity of contraction; automaticity increased by increasing rate of slow diastolic (phase 4) depolarization. Reflex vagal slowing of HR can oppose direct effects of NE and result in decreased output even though force and stroke volume is increased.

2. Epinephrine (EPI): endogenous catecholamine in adrenal medulla.
   a. About 90% of catecholamine released from adrenal medulla; is a hormone; acts strongly on all alpha- and beta-adrenoceptors by a direct action; not effective orally; causes metabolic actions seen in fight or flight response.
   b. EPI stimulates both alpha- and beta$_2$-adrenoceptors in blood vessels; with small doses or with slow infusion, get vasodilation (skeletal muscle) and diastolic BP decreases (beta$_2$ effect); with larger doses, get vasoconstriction (skin and splanchnics) and TPR is increased (alpha effect); veins are constricted. EPI often added to local anesthetic preparations for local vasoconstriction (best in skin which has few non-innervated beta$_2$-adrenoceptors).
   c. Direct effect on beta$_1$ receptor of heart - like NE; increased rate (automaticity), force and cardiac output; with large doses acts like NE to cause reflex vagal slowing and decreased output despite direct effects.
   d. Used to treat anaphylaxis (parenterally), bronchospasm (sub Q) and topically for minor bleeding.

3. Isoproterenol: synthetic nonselective beta-adrenoceptor stimulant.
   a. Also catecholamine; acts directly on all beta-adrenoceptors; no alpha action; not effective orally; used in treatment of asthma (beta$_2$) and experimentally in cardiogenic shock (beta$_1$).
   b. Stimulates beta$_2$-adrenoceptors of blood vessels to cause vasodilation - decreased diastolic BP and TPR.
   c. Direct beta$_1$ receptor stimulation in heart to increase rate, force and output; no reflex vagal activation.

4. Dopamine (DA):
   a. Catecholamine; precursor in formation of NE and EPI in peripheral autonomic system; acts as CNS neurotransmitter especially in extrapyramidal motor system.
   b. Not orally effective; DA acts on alpha- and beta$_1$-adrenoceptors to increase BP and HR; also causes vasodilation of renal vasculature by action on "dopamine receptors".
   c. Sometimes used in treatment of patients with shock primarily for cardiac and renal actions.
   d. Replacement in CNS by giving precursor (-DOPA) is a treatment to relieve the symptoms of Parkinson's disease.

D. SYMPATHOMIMETICS (Non-catecholamines) - May exert effects by direct or indirect actions. <u>Direct</u> sympathomimetics act to stimulate <u>alpha</u>- or <u>beta</u>-adrenoceptors. <u>Indirect</u> sympathomimetics may release stored NE from nerve terminals or may block reuptake mechanism (many do both). <u>Tricyclic Antidepressants</u> act like <u>cocaine</u> in preventing reuptake of catecholamines into nerve terminals. <u>Reuptake</u> is principle mechanism for termination of the actions of NE.

1. <u>Tyramine</u>: indirect actions only - effects produced by the release of endogenous norepinephrine from storage granules; will be ineffective if pretreated with reserpine or chronically with guanethidine. Found in foods such as wine, cheese, beer, etc. but is normally broken down by MAO in gut and liver (no <u>alpha</u>-carbon CH_3). Tyramine in foods can lead to hypertensive crisis in patients on MAO inhibitor drugs such as tranylcypromine; cardiovascular effects on heart and blood vessels produced by the NE released.

2 & 3.   <u>Amphetamine</u> and <u>Methamphetamine</u>: indirect acting (primarily releases endogenous NE). Orally effective due to <u>alpha</u> carbon CH_3 group. Potent CNS effects. Tolerance readily develops to appetite suppressive and mood elevating effects. Causes syndrome resembling paranoia in repeated large doses; only slight direct action on peripheral <u>alpha</u> receptors. Acidification of urine aids in renal elimination.

4. <u>Phenylpropanolamine</u>: many actions same as amphetamine; orally effective; long term anorexiant action questionable; occasional use as nasal decongestant. Note that drugs that are without 3- or 4-OH on ring and with CH_3 on <u>alpha</u>-carbon are refractory to breakdown by MAO and COMT.

5. <u>Ephedrine</u>: mixed actions (direct and indirect) acts like epinephrine on both <u>alpha</u>- and <u>beta</u>-adrenoceptors; orally effective; one of most commonly used sympathomimetics; increases BP, heart rate and contractility; bronchial muscle relaxation; mydriasis without cycloplegia; nasal decongestion.

6. <u>Metaraminol</u>: mixed acting; more direct than indirect and mainly acts on <u>alpha</u> receptors. May cause hypotension if given over long periods of time as it is taken into nerve terminals where it can serve as a false transmitter. Used to elevate BP in hypotensive states.

7. <u>Phenylephrine</u>: direct acting - primarily on <u>alpha</u>-adrenoceptors; oral dose much greater than i.v. or i.m. dose; widely used as nasal decongestant but can lead to more congestion <u>via</u> irritant actions on nasal mucosa (rebound phenomena); produces vasoconstriction with minimal cardiac effects. Sometimes used to treat atrial tachycardia.

8. <u>Methoxamine</u>: direct acting - like phenylephrine; vasoconstrictor; almost pure <u>alpha</u>-adrenoceptor stimulant with minimal cardiac effects; may use to treat atrial tachycardia due to baroreceptor reflex effects; no significant CNS effects.

9. <u>Metaproterenol</u>: direct acting; "selective" <u>beta$_2$</u>-adrenoceptor agonist; used as bronchodilator with minimal cardiac actions; orally effective (resistant to COMT); sometimes used to inhibit uterus in premature labor.

10. <u>Terbutaline</u>: direct acting; also "selective" <u>beta</u>$_2$-adrenoceptor agonist; used as bronchodilator; uses and actions similar to metaproterenol. Oral, s.c. or inhalation, longer acting than metaproterenol but more cardiac effects.
11. <u>Albuterol</u>: similar indications to terbutaline; inhalation or oral; duration similar to metaproterenol; few CV effects.
12. <u>Ritodrine</u>: <u>Beta</u>$_2$-adrenoceptor selective; developed as a uterine relaxant; 30% absorbed by oral route; administered also IV and IM.
13. <u>Dobutamine</u>: direct acting; "selective" <u>beta</u>$_1$-adrenoceptor agonist; used to increase heart rate and contractility; increases myocardial contractile force more than HR; short acting and not orally effective; given as i.v. infusion. Used to treat severe congestive heart failure.

STRUCTURES AND MAIN CLINICAL USES OF SOME IMPORTANT SYMPATHOMIMETIC DRUGS

		β CH	α CH	NH	ACTION	α-RECEPTOR A,N,P,V	β-RECEPTOR B,C	CNS
Phenylethylamine		H	H	H				
Epinephrine	3-OH, 4-OH	OH	H	CH$_3$	DIRECT	A,P,V	B,C	
Norepinephrine	3-OH, 4-OH	OH	H	H	DIRECT	P		
Isoproterenol	3-OH, 4-OH	OH	H	CH(CH$_3$)$_2$	DIRECT		B,C	
Dopamine	3-OH, 4-OH	H	H	H	DIRECT	P	C	CNS
Tyramine	4-OH	H	H	H	INDIRECT			
Amphetamine		H	CH$_3$	H	INDIRECT			CNS
Phenylpropanolamine		OH	CH$_3$	H	INDIRECT			CNS
Methamphetamine		H	CH$_3$	CH$_3$	INDIRECT	P		CNS
Ephedrine		OH	CH$_3$	CH$_3$	MIXED	N,P	B,C	
Metaraminol	3-OH	OH	CH$_3$	H	DIRECT	P		
Phenylephrine	3-OH	OH	H	CH$_3$	DIRECT	N,P		
Methoxamine	2-OCH$_3$, 5-OCH$_3$	OH	CH$_3$	H	DIRECT	P		
Metaproterenol	3-OH, 5-OH	OH	H	CH(CH$_3$)$_2$	DIRECT		B	
Terbutaline	3-OH, 5-OH	OH	H	C(CH$_3$)$_3$	DIRECT		B	
Albuterol	3-CH$_2$OH, 4-OH	OH	H	C(CH$_3$)$_3$	DIRECT		B	
Ritodrine	4-OH	OH	CH$_3$	1	DIRECT		U,B	
Dobutamine	3-OH, 4-OH	H	H	2	DIRECT		C	

A: Allergic reactions
N: Nasal decongestion
P: Pressor (may include action)
V: Local vasoconstriction (e.g. in local anesthetics)
B: Bronchodilator
C: Cardiac
U: Uterine relaxant
CNS: Central nervous system

E. DRUGS INHIBITING SYMPATHETIC FUNCTION (Sympatholytics)

1. <u>False Transmitter Precursors</u>:
   a. <u>Alpha methyl meta tyrosine</u> → metaraminol (false transmitter)
   b. <u>Alpha methyl dopa</u> → <u>alpha methyl NE</u> (CNS action in treating hypertension; like clonidine).

2. <u>Adrenergic Neuron Inhibitors</u>:
   a. <u>Reserpine</u>: prevents storage and thus causes depletion of neuronal NE. Also depletes stores of epinephrine, dopamine and serotonin; CNS effects include sedation; used to treat hypertension.
   b. <u>Guanethidine</u>: blocks nerve action potentials at fine terminals (also has many other actions including reserpine-like depletion of monoamines). Effective and potent antihypertensive drug; orally effective; does not act on CNS; chronic administration depletes <u>peripheral</u> catecholamines but not those in CNS. Taken up by nerve endings, thus effect blocked by reuptake inhibitors (tricyclic antidepressants and cocaine).

3. <u>Alpha-adrenoceptor Blockers</u>: side effects include postural hypotension (orthostatic), reflex tachycardia, miosis, nasal stuffiness, inhibition of ejaculation.
   a. <u>Phenoxybenzamine</u>: antagonism of <u>alpha</u>-adrenoceptors (mainly <u>alpha</u>$_1$); blocks vasoconstriction caused by nerve stimulation or sympathomimetic drugs; produces fall in BP by reducing sympathetic tone, but get tachycardia because <u>beta</u>-adrenoceptors not blocked; causes EPI "reversal" - converts a pressor response to EPI to a depressor response (no effect on cardiostimulation to EPI); longer acting agent; first competitive then becomes noncompetitive. Used during treatment of pheochromocytoma.
   b. <u>Phentolamine</u>: short acting only due to competitive blockade of <u>alpha</u>-adrenoceptors; in past, used in diagnosis of pheochromocytoma; used to block excessive pressor rise caused by catecholamines released by pheochromocytoma during surgical removal; blocks <u>alpha</u>$_1$- and <u>alpha</u>$_2$-adrenoceptors.
   c. <u>Prazosin</u>: used in treatment of hypertension, probably due to blockade of peripheral <u>alpha</u>$_1$-adrenoceptors; may have some direct vasodilator action; less reflex tachycardia observed which may be due to CNS effect to decrease sympathetic tone. "First dose" hypotensive effect; administer slowly.
   d. <u>Yohimbine</u>: "selective" antagonist for <u>alpha</u>$_2$-adrenoceptors; experimentally shown to antagonize CNS hypotensive actions of clonidine and <u>alpha</u>-methyl-DOPA.

4. <u>Beta-Adrenoceptor Blockers</u>: used to treat hypertension, angina, cardiac arrhythmias, reduce incidence of myocardial reinfarction and for glaucoma. Also to treat peripheral effects of hyperthyroidism and prophylactic for migraine headache. Caution in patients with congestive heart failure, bronchial asthma, or diabetes.

a. <u>Propranolol</u>: nonselective <u>beta</u> receptor antagonist (blocks both beta$_1$- and beta$_2$-adrenoceptors); orally effective; t½ = 3-5 hrs., first-pass hepatic metabolism seen particularly with the initial dose; 90% bound to plasma proteins; has a local anesthetic ("quinidine-like") action; used in treating cardiac arrhythmias and in treating hypertension. Use with caution especially in patients with heart disease, asthma and diabetes (may mask the tachycardia "sign" of hypoglycemia in diabetics taking insulin).

b. <u>Metoprolol</u>: cardioselective beta$_1$-adrenoceptor antagonist (50X more potent for beta$_1$); like propranolol, subject to first-pass metabolic breakdown by liver; only slight membrane stabilizing action; 10% bound to plasma proteins; less effect on bronchial smooth muscle; more CNS side effects.

c. <u>Atenolol</u>: Also cardioselective (beta$_1$); longer half life (6-9 hrs) thus fewer doses needed; renal excretion; less hypoglycemia and less CNS effects.

d. <u>Pindolol</u>: nonselective; hepatic and renal elimination; intrinsic sympathomimetic activity (ISA) may contribute to less depression of HR and CO at rest.

e. <u>Nadolol</u>: also nonselective <u>beta</u>-adrenoceptor antagonist; longer acting than propranolol (t½ = 20-24 hrs), thus suitable for once per day administration; no significant local anesthetic or "quinidine-like" action; no ISA; excluded from CNS.

f. <u>Timolol</u>: non-selective <u>beta</u>-adrenoceptor antagonist; no significant local anesthetic or "quinidine-like" action; 5 to 10X as potent as propranolol; a drug of choice given topically to treat open angle glaucoma (reduces formation of aqueous humor); also used post-myocardial infarction.

g. <u>Betaxolol</u>: also used as <u>beta</u>-adrenoceptor blocker to treat glaucoma; beta$_1$ selective.

h. <u>Esmolol</u>: cardioselective ultra-short half-life due to rapid metabolism (about 10 min); used i.v. for control of emergency ventricular arrhythmias.

5. <u>Mixed Antagonist</u>:
   a. <u>Labetalol</u>: alpha$_1$ antagonist; nonselective <u>beta</u> antagonist; some beta$_2$-adrenoceptor stimulation. Oral or i.v.; t½ about 5 hrs; decreases plasma renin. Used to treat hypertension and sometimes clonidine withdrawal syndrome. Postural hypotension (<u>alpha</u>) and other side effects as with <u>beta</u>-adrenoceptor antagonists.

REVIEW QUESTIONS

ONE BEST ANSWER

1. Which of the following agents most likely would be used for treatment of urinary retention?

   A. Atropine
   B. Acetylcholine
   C. Hexamethonium
   D. Methacholine
   E. Bethanechol

2. Acetylcholine is the normal neurotransmitter at all of the followings sites **EXCEPT**:

   A. Nerve endings to the adrenal medulla
   B. Sympathetic ganglia
   C. Neuromuscular junction
   D. Parasympathetic ganglia
   E. Sympathetic neuroeffector junction

3. Which one of the following classes of drugs would be expected to produce miosis and cycloplegia when applied topically to the eye?

   A. Ganglionic blocking drugs
   B. Muscarinic stimulating drugs
   C. α-Adrenoceptor blockers
   D. ß-Adrenoceptor blockers
   E. None of the above

4. The reflex change in heart rate in response to norepinephrine, given intravenously to a dog, would be enhanced by prior injection of:

   A. Ganglionic blocking drugs
   B. Muscarinic receptor blocking drugs
   C. α-Adrenoceptor blocking drugs
   D. Applies to all of the above
   E. Does not apply to any of the above

5. A patient who has "spasms of accommodation", miosis, increased gut motility, excessive salivation, and increased sweating may have been given a therapeutic dose of which one of the following?

   A. A ganglionic blocking drug
   B. A muscarinic blocking drug
   C. An anticholinesterase drug
   D. A ß-adrenergic blocking drug
   E. An α-adrenergic blocking drug

6. The effects of which one of the following drugs are terminated by spontaneous, non-enzymatic hydrolysis at physiological pH?

   A. Labetalol
   B. Succinylcholine
   C. Vecuronium
   D. Pancuronium
   E. Atracurium

7. Administration of neostigmine might potentiate the neuromuscular blockade produced by which of the following agents?

   A. Succinylcholine
   B. Pancuronium
   C. Gallamine
   D. d-Tubocurarine
   E. Hemicholinium

8. Stimulation of the vagus nerve in the neck will slow the heart rate directly. Which of the following drugs would inhibit this response to vagal stimulation?

   A. Atropine
   B. Pilocarpine
   C. Neostigmine
   D. Bethanechol
   E. Methacholine

9. Which one of the following drugs produces an antihypertensive response which is reversed by administration of yohimbine?

   A. Metoprolol
   B. Clonidine
   C. Dobutamine
   D. Metaproterenol
   E. Nadolol

10. Which one of the following is a drug of choice in the treatment of "wide angle" glaucoma?

    A. Nadolol
    B. Propranolol
    C. Prazosin
    D. Yohimbine
    E. Timolol

38

ONE BEST ANSWER

11. Which one of the following is the primary metabolic product of norepinephrine found in the brain?

A. VMA
B. 3-Methoxy-4-hydroxy-mandelic acid
C. 3-Methoxy-4-hydroxy-phenylglycol
D. α-Methyl norepinephrine
E. α-Phenylethanolamine

12. Which one of the following drugs most likely would be expected to produce tachycardia, orthostatic hypotension and inhibition of ejaculation?

A. Reserpine
B. Amphetamine
C. Metoprolol
D. Phenoxybenzamine
E. Propranolol

13. The vascular response following intravenous administration of all of the following agents would be of less magnitude after reserpine pretreatment **EXCEPT**:

A. Methamphetamine
B. Ephedrine
C. Prazosin
D. Methoxamine
E. Tyramine

14. An anesthetized dog is premedicated with propranolol and atropine. An intravenous dose of norepinephrine would then produce which one of the following groups of responses?

A. Increase in arterial blood pressure, relaxation of smooth muscle of the G.I. tract, contraction of the radial muscle of the iris.
B. Increase in blood pressure, increase in heart rate, relaxation of radial muscle of the iris.
C. Decrease in blood pressure, relaxation of smooth muscle of the G.I. tract.
D. No change in heart rate, no change in blood pressure, no change in radial muscle tone.
E. Decrease in arterial blood pressure, no change in heart rate.

15. Propranolol most likely would be contraindicated in the treatment of which one of the following conditions?

A. Glaucoma
B. Asthma
C. Nasal congestion
D. Hypertension
E. Myasthenia gravis

16. All of the following statements are true of the actions of prazosin **EXCEPT**:

A. Lowers systemic blood pressure
B. Blocks pressor response to norepinephrine
C. Acts as an indirect acting sympathomimetic
D. Produces only a modest reflex tachycardia
E. "Selective" for α_1 adrenergic receptors

17. Which one of the following drugs acts primarily to inhibit reuptake of norepinephrine?

A. Tyramine
B. Pargyline
C. Imipramine
D. Prazosin
E. Ritodrine

18. All of the following are potent agonists for β_1-adrenoceptors **EXCEPT**:

A. Epinephrine
B. Dobutamine
C. Isoproterenol
D. Norepinephrine
E. Metoprolol

ONE BEST ANSWER

19. Intravenous administration of Drug X to an anesthetized dog produces a vasodepressor response. After administration of Drug Y, Drug X produces no change in pressure. Which of the following pairs of drugs would NOT produce the above sequence of events?

Drug X could be: Drug Y could be:

   A. Isoproterenol   Nadolol
   B. Methacholine   Atropine
   C. Isoproterenol   Scopolamine
   D. Muscarine   Atropine
   E. Isoproterenol   Propranolol

20. Of the following drugs which one would be most useful in the treatment of paroxysmal atrial tachycardia due to reflex effects?

   A. Pilocarpine
   B. Epinephrine
   C. Atropine
   D. Phenylephrine
   E. Propranolol

21. All of the following are classified as "direct acting" sympathomimetic amines EXCEPT:

   A. Ritodrine
   B. Amphetamine
   C. Albuterol
   D. Methoxamine
   E. Dobutamine

22. Which one of the following drugs produces a systemic cardiovascular response after oral administration?

   A. Norepinephrine
   B. Epinephrine
   C. Hexamethonium
   D. Isoproterenol
   E. Ephedrine

23. Epinephrine may cause all of the following EXCEPT:

   A. Increase in cardiac output
   B. Increase in coronary blood flow
   C. Stimulation of the central nervous system
   D. Breakdown of muscle glycogen
   E. Bronchiolar constriction

24. Epinephrine is useful as an adjuvant for local anesthesia of cutaneous regions BECAUSE:

   A. Epinephrine's main influence in the body is metabolic (i.e. causes breakdown of glucose which aids in healing of wounds).
   B. Cutaneous vascular smooth muscle has many α-adrenoceptors but only a few β_2-adrenoceptors.
   C. Epinephrine has a potent effect on α-adrenoceptors but only a weak action on β-adrenoceptors.
   D. Epinephrine also has a potent anti-bacterial action.
   E. Non-innervated vascular muscarinic receptors are not stimulated by epinephrine.

25. Which of the following combinations of agents would be necessary to block the cardiovascular effects produced by the injection of an indirectly acting sympathomimetic drug?

   A. Atropine and phenoxybenzamine
   B. Atropine and propranolol
   C. Phenoxybenzamine and propranolol
   D. Phenoxybenzamine and curare
   E. Amphetamine and propranolol

26. All of the following compounds are precursors of norepinephrine and epinephrine EXCEPT:

   A. 3,4 Dihydroxyphenylethylamine (dopamine)
   B. Phenylalanine
   C. Tyrosine
   D. 3,4 Dihydroxyphenylalanine (DOPA)
   E. 3-Methoxy, 4-hydroxy mandelic acid (VMA)

ONE BEST ANSWER

27. Adrenergic ß receptors subserve all of the following actions **EXCEPT**:

    A. Vasodilation
    B. Bronchodilation
    C. Increased myocardial contractile force
    D. Contraction of the radial muscle of the iris
    E. Increased heart rate

28. With which of the following conditions would atropine most likely be contraindicated?

    A. Myasthenia gravis
    B. Asthma
    C. Glaucoma
    D. Nasal congestion
    E. Hypertension

29. In a patient receiving atropine, norepinephrine produces an increased blood pressure and heart rate. After this patient has been given an unknown drug, the administration of norepinephrine now produces about the same increase in heart rate as it did previously but a smaller increase in blood pressure. The unknown drug could be:

    A. Reserpine
    B. Propranolol
    C. Guanethidine
    D. Prazosin
    E. Hexamethonium

30. The therapeutic effectiveness of neostigmine in myasthenia gravis is thought to be due to:

    A. Its ability to protect the muscle endplate against acetylcholine
    B. Its ability to increase the rate of synthesis of acetylcholine
    C. Its ability to inactivate cholinesterase
    D. Its stimulant action on the motor nerve terminals at the motor endplate

31. Profound skeletal muscle paralysis develops in a patient after he is given a dose of tubocurarine which ordinarily does not produce detectable paralysis. What condition is this patient most likely to have?

    A. Myotonia congenita
    B. Myasthenia gravis
    C. Multiple sclerosis
    D. Atypical pseudocholinesterase
    E. None of the above

32. Pilocarpine most likely would be administered to a patient being treated for:

    A. Myasthenia gravis
    B. Glaucoma
    C. Hypertension
    D. Orthostatic hypotension
    E. Congestive heart failure

33. Low concentrations of sympathomimetic agents which are ineffective in the normal individual might produce a hypertensive response in a person treated chronically with which one of the following drugs?

    A. Tyramine
    B. Atropine
    C. Guanethidine
    D. Propranolol
    E. Phentolamine

34. An anesthetized dog is pretreated with scopolamine and phentolamine. Intravenous administration of carbachol might be expected to produce a(n) ___ in blood pressure:

    A. Increase
    B. Decrease
    C. No change

35. In the question above, the firing rate of the postganglionic nerves would ___ in response to carbachol:

    A. Increase
    B. Decrease
    C. Not change

ONE BEST ANSWER

36. The drug of first choice in the emergency treatment of anaphylactic shock is:

A. Epinephrine
B. Norepinephrine
C. Cortisone
D. Diphenhydramine
E. Atropine

37. Dobutamine:

A. Produces dilation of renal blood vessels
B. Is effective orally
C. Is refractory to inactivation by MAO
D. Is useful primarily as a beta₁ receptor agonist
E. Produces its effects by an indirect action

* * * * * * * * * *

MATCHING

A. Neostigmine
B. Hexamethonium
C. Edrophonium
D. Atropine
E. Succinylcholine

38. Tachycardia, anhidrosis; xerostomia; hypotension; constipation

39. Mydriasis, cycloplegia, anhidrosis; tachycardia; CNS excitation

* * * * * * * * * *

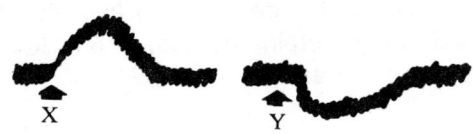

A. X same, Y reduced
B. X reduced, Y reduced
C. X enhanced, Y enhanced
D. X enhanced, Y reduced
E. X same, Y same

40. If (in reference to the blood pressure tracings above) drug X is epinephrine and drug Y is isoproterenol, then after nadolol you would expect:

41. If (in reference to the blood pressure tracings above) drug X is epinephrine and drug Y is isoproterenol, then after hexamethonium you would expect?

* * * * * * * * * *

MATCHING

A. Edrophonium
B. Pilocarpine
C. Atropine
D. Physostigmine
E. Neostigmine

42. Most rational treatment for atropine poisoning

43. Useful in the diagnosis of myasthenia gravis because of its short duration of action

44. Drug of choice for treatment of myasthenia gravis

45. Inhibits salivary secretion

42

MATCHING

The following tracings represent changes in blood pressure in response to intravenous administration of drugs I, II and III before (Control) and after treatment with reserpine (reserpine treated). From the list below identify drugs I, II and III.

    A. Tyramine
    B. Methoxamine
    C. Ritodrine
    D. Ephedrine
    E. Metaproterenol

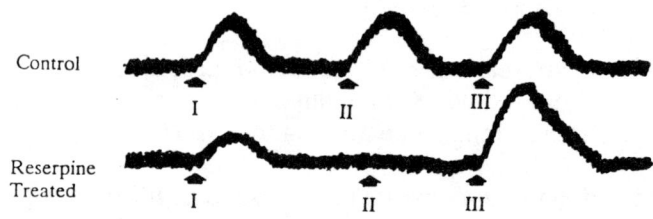

46. Drug I

47. Drug II

48. Drug III

MATCHING: Use each letter only once

    A. Nadolol
    B. Timolol
    C. Metoprolol
    D. Atenolol
    E. Pindolol

49. Long half-life (20-24hr) allows once/day administration

50. "Cardio-selective"; primarily hepatic elimination

51. Has intrinsic sympathomimetic activity (ISA)

52. "Cardio-selective"; primarily renal elimination

53. Drug of choice for open angle glaucoma

* * * * * * * * *

MATCHING

    A. Metoprolol   F. Methylnorepinephrine
    B. Metanephrine   G. Methamphetamine
    C. Metaproterenol   H. Methacholine
    D. Metaraminol   I. Muscarine
    E. Methyldopa   J. Monoamine oxidase

54. "False transmitter" formed from α-methyl-meta-tyrosine; sympathomimetic

55. Releases stored monoamines from nerve terminals

56. Metabolite formed by action of COMT on epinephrine

57. Converted in CNS to an antihypertensive metabolite with clonidine-like action

58. Associated with mitochondria in nerve ending

59. Active metabolite of methyldopa

60. "Selective" β_2 stimulant (agonist)

61. Alkaloid with vasodilating actions

62. "Cardioselective" adrenergic blocking drug

63. Produces atropine-sensitive vasodilation; synthetic compound

MATCHING

An answer may be used more than once.

In a dog anesthetized with pentobarbital, recording electrodes are placed on:

  I Carotid sinus baroreceptor nerve fibers
 II Splanchnic (sympathetic) nerve fibers (preganglionic)
III Inferior cardiac (sympathetic) nerve fibers (postganglionic)
IV Vagal (parasympathetic) nerve fibers

What changes (if any) in firing rates would be expected to occur following the administration of the last drug in each series of drugs listed below? Presume that sufficient time for the actions of the premedicating agents has been allowed and then the last agent is given intravenously.

Give one answer for each set of nerves (in order I-IV) from the choices below. ↑ = increase of nerve activity; ↓ = decrease nerve activity; ↔ = no change in neural firing.

	I	II	III	IV
A.	↔	↔	↔	↔
B.	↑	↓	↓	↑
C.	↔	↓	↓	↑
D.	↓	↑	↑	↓
E.	↑	↓	↔	↑

64. Propranolol, and atropine; then phenylephrine

65. Propranolol, atropine and reserpine; then phenylephrine

66. Propranolol, atropine, reserpine and hexamethonium; then phenylephrine

67. Propranolol, atropine, reserpine, hexamethonium and phenoxybenzamine; then phenylephrine

68. What changes (if any) would be expected in the firing rates in the above four nerves following bilateral common carotid artery occlusion in an animal that had been pretreated with atropine, phentolamine and propranolol

MATCHING

The following tracings represent the changes in mean systemic blood pressure in an anesthetized dog in response to drugs A, B, C and D given intravenously. The first panel shows the control responses, the second panel shows the responses after reserpine pretreatment. The last panel shows the responses after <u>subsequent</u> administration of atropine. The same dose of each agent is given in each case.

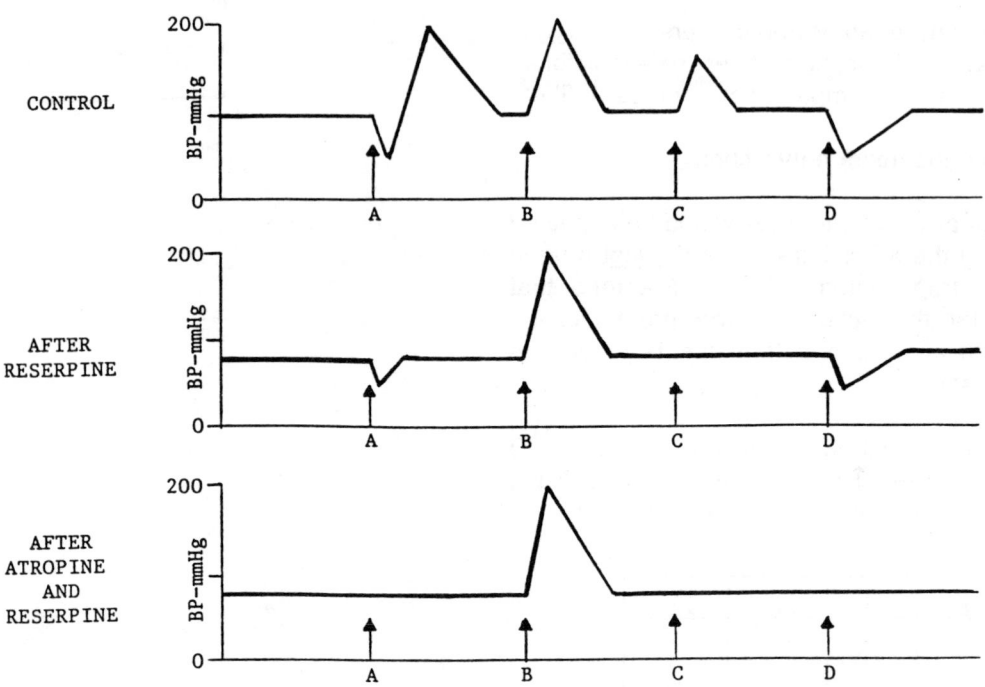

From the above information what are drugs A - D?

69. Drug A is:

    A. Nicotine
    B. Hexamethonium
    C. Trimethaphan
    D. Ephedrine
    E. Norepinephrine

70. Drug B is:

    A. Nicotine
    B. Histamine
    C. Ephedrine
    D. Isoproterenol
    E. Phenylephrine

71. Drug C is:

    A. Norepinephrine
    B. Tyramine
    C. Epinephrine
    D. Phenylephrine
    E. Isoproterenol

72. Drug D is:

    A. Tyramine
    B. Ephedrine
    C. Pilocarpine
    D. Phenylephrine
    E. Histamine

MATCHING

The following bar graphs represent changes in blood pressure measured in an anesthetized dog. (+) equals an increase and (-) equals a decrease in blood pressure in response to intravenous administration of drugs A-D. The first series of responses are controls (no pretreatment). The second, third, fourth and fifth series are responses to the same drugs following pretreatment of the agents P-S administered sequentially. Regard the effect of the pretreatment as being complete and lasting throughout the experiment. Identify unknown drugs A-D and each pretreatment or blocker P-S.

Drugs (A-D)	Pretreatment (P-S)
A. Acetylcholine (100 µg/kg)	A. Atropine
B. Methacholine	B. Reserpine
C. Tyramine	C. Phenoxybenzamine
D. Norepinephrine	D. Hexamethonium
E. Angiotensin	E. Propranolol

73. Drug A:

74. Drug B:

75. Drug C:

76. Drug D:

77. Pretreatment P:

78. Pretreatment Q:

79. Pretreatment R:

80. Pretreatment S:

CHAPTER 3: <u>DRUGS ACTING ON THE KIDNEY</u>

I. DIURETICS

A. RENAL TRANSPORT SYSTEMS

1. PROXIMAL CONVOLUTED TUBULE

Approximately 60 - 70 % of the filtered sodium and potassium ions are removed **isotonically** from the proximal tubule. After passing the length of the proximal tubule, the volume of the filtrate has therefore been reduced by 30 - 40 %, without altering sodium and potassium ion concentrations. Actively transported species include:

>   sodium
>   potassium
>   bicarbonate

Glucose and amino acids are completely reabsorbed in the proximal tubule. If sodium and potassium ion reabsorption are inhibited at this site, the transport mechanisms remaining in the nephron (loop of Henle and distal convoluted tubule) can fully compensate and the final urine composition is not altered. Bicarbonate reabsorption and urine pH are primarily controlled in the proximal tubule.

2. ASCENDING LOOP OF HENLE

Approximately 15 - 20 % of the total filtered sodium and chloride load are reabsorbed at this site. Chloride is the actively transported species. Sodium and potassium reabsorption are passive processes.

3. DISTAL CONVOLUTED TUBULE

8 - 10 % of the sodium and potassium load is reabsorbed in the distal convoluted tubule. Active transport mechanisms are present in the distal convoluted tubule for:

>   sodium
>   potassium
>   chloride

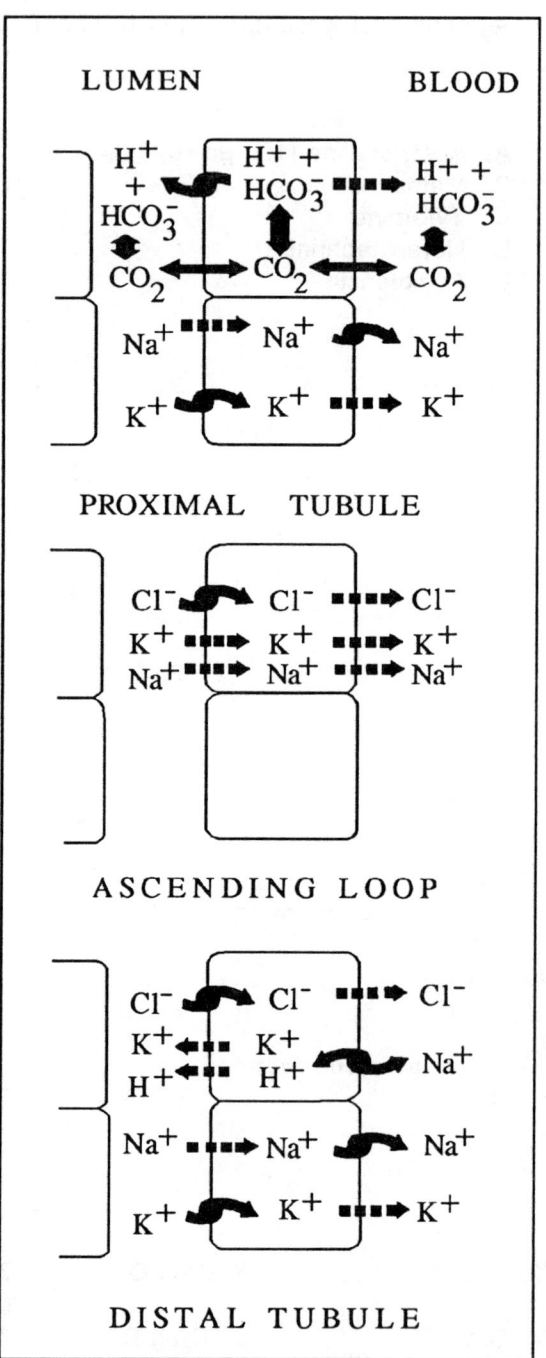

Co-transport or exchange transport mechanisms exist in the distal convoluted tubule for

> sodium and hydrogen ion
> sodium and potassium.

Sodium-potassium exchange and to some extent, sodium-hydrogen ion exchange are controlled by aldosterone and urine sodium concentrations. When the sodium concentrations increase in the distal tubule, sodium ions are absorbed in exchange for potassium ion/hydrogen ion excretion. Increased aldosterone thus increases sodium ion retention in plasma and urinary potassium excretion. There is a resultant decrease in urine pH (H+ ion excretion in urine).

B. DIURETIC DRUG CLASSES

1. OSMOTIC DIURETICS

The mechanism of action of the osmotic diuretics is based upon the drugs:

a. Being freely filtered by the glomerulus,
b. Undergoing no reabsorption from the glomerular filtrate, and
c. Producing increased plasma and subsequently, urine osmolarity.

Examples: mannitol (prototype)

Toxicity: The drug can produce fluid overload with inadequate glomerular filtration.

Mannitol can only be administered intravenously. Mannitol is not absorbed with oral administration and produces severe diarrhea. The drugs produce diuresis (increased urine flow) without natruresis (increased sodium ion excretion) and **are therefore ineffective for the mobilization of edema fluid**.

Therapeutic Uses: a. Acute reduction of cerebrospinal or intraocular pressure
b. Evaluation of acute oliguria - prevent anuria
c. Acute poisonings - dilution of toxin in urine by increasing urinary flow

2. CARBONIC ANHYDRASE INHIBITORS

Carbonic anhydrase inhibitors reduce the absorption of bicarbonate ions from the glomerular filtrate in the proximal convoluted tubule. A 90 % or greater inhibition of carbonic anhydrase activity must be observed before significant diuresis is observed. Both diuresis and natruresis are limited as the increased excretion of bicarbonate in the urine quickly depletes plasma bicarbonate. The carbonic anhydrase inhibitors are primarily used in the treatment of glaucoma as inhibitors of aqueous humor formation.

<u>Examples</u>: acetazolamide (prototype)

<u>Toxicity</u>: drowsiness

<u>Therapeutic Uses</u>: a. Alkalinization of urine - compensatory metabolic acidosis
                               b. Treatment of glaucoma - decreased aqueous humor formation

3. HIGH CEILING or LOOP DIURETICS

The loop diuretics are actively secreted into the proximal convoluted tubule from plasma and act upon the ascending loop of Henle to inhibit the reabsorption of chloride from the tubular lumen. <u>The loop diuretics are the most effective natriuretic and diuretic agents available. The drugs increase sodium and potassium excretion, and increase urine volume.</u> Diuresis is independent of acid-base balance and has a rapid onset of action (within 10 - 20 minutes following IV administration). The drugs also increase calcium ion excretion into the urine.

<u>Examples</u>: furosemide (LASIX) (prototype)
                        bumetanide
                        ethacrynic acid

<u>Toxicity</u>: a. Allergic reactions - The drugs are related to the antibacterial sulfonamides
                       b. Hypokalemia, dehydration - can potentiate digitalis toxicity and precipitate skeletal muscle weakness
                       c. Hyperuricemia - excretion of drugs in proximal convoluted tubules interferes with uric acid excretion. May precipitate gouty arthritis.

<u>Therapeutic Uses</u>: a. Treatment of congestive heart failure - reduces circulating plasma volume by natruresis (increased sodium excretion) and diuresis (increased urine volume)
                               b. Treatment of acute oliguria - prevent anuria by maintaining urine formation

4. THIAZIDE DIURETICS

The thiazide diuretics are actively secreted into the proximal convoluted tubule and inhibit sodium ion reabsorption in the distal convoluted tubule. Calcium ion excretion in the urine is decreased. The thiazide diuretics are weak inhibitors of carbonic anhydrase, but diuresis is <u>not</u> dependent upon an inhibition of carbonic anhydrase. Incomplete inhibition of carbonic anhydrase does produce a small increase in urine pH. The drugs may also decrease glomerular filtration is some patients and may therefore aggravate existing mild renal failure. All 100 or more thiazide diuretics share a common mechanism of action and common side effects. They differ from each other only in potency and duration of action.

<u>Examples:</u>   chlorothiazide
               hydrochlorothiazide (prototype)
               chlorthalidone (not chemically a thiazide, same mechanism of action)

<u>Toxicity:</u>
a. Renal failure - due to decreased glomerular filtration rate
b. Hyperuricemia - may precipitate gouty arthritis
c. Hypokalemia - muscle weakness, potentiates digitalis toxicity
d. Hyperglycemia - decreased glucose tolerance
e. Hypercholesterolemia, hypertriglyceridemia - mild effect

<u>Therapeutic Uses:</u>
a. Treatment of hypertension - used alone or with other agents to reduce compensatory sodium/water retention
b. Mild diuresis - loop diuretics used more commonly for the treatment of heart failure

5. ALDOSTERONE ANTAGONISTS, CONVERTING ENZYME INHIBITORS, AND POTASSIUM SPARING DIURETICS

Renin is an enzyme release by specialized cells of the proximal convoluted tubule. The enzyme cleaves the inactive peptide angiotensinogen into angiotensin I. Angiotensin I is then further acted upon by angiotensin converting enzyme in the lung to produce angiotensin II. Angiotensin II is a vasoconstrictor and stimulates aldosterone release from the adrenal cortex. The renin-angiotensin mechanism for aldosterone release is dependent upon the actions of both renin and converting enzyme for the activation of angiotensinogen. Under conditions of (1) low plasma sodium concentrations and/or (2) increased sympathetic nervous system stimulation, increased quantities of renin are released by the kidney into the systemic circulation.

Aldosterone is secreted from the adrenal cortex and plays an important role in the control of renal sodium excretion and extracellular electrolyte balance. The hormone acts to:
(1) Stimulate sodium reabsorption,
(2) Stimulate sodium-potassium exchange in the distal tubule, and
(3) Stimulate hydrogen ion secretion in the proximal tubule.

The net results of the actions of aldosterone are (1) sodium ion retention, (2) an increased potassium ion excretion, and (3) mild systemic alkalosis.

ALDOSTERONE ANTAGONISTS - Spironolactone (prototype)

ANGIOTENSIN CONVERTING ENZYME INHIBITORS - Captopril (prototype), lisinopril, ramipril, and enalapril are inhibitors of angiotensin converting enzyme (ACE) in the lung and prevent the activation of angiotensin I to angiotensin II. Because ACE inhibitors prevent activation of angiotensin II from angiotensin I, they prevent the direct effects of angiotensin II upon blood vessels (vasoconstriction) as well as preventing aldosterone release from the adrenal cortex. As antihypertensive agents, the ACE inhibitors are more effective than spironolactone.

POTASSIUM SPARING DIURETICS - Triamterene and amiloride directly interfere with sodium transport in the distal convoluted tubule. Although the drugs do not act upon the renin-angiotensin axis, the net effect upon urinary composition is similar.

Toxicities:　a. hyperkalemia - do not use potassium sparing diuretics and potassium supplements together
b. dysgeusia - disturbance or loss of sense of taste (captopril only)
c. hypotension (ACE inhibitors)

Therapeutic Uses:　a. Potassium retention (combined with other diuretics)
b. Hypertension and heart failure (ACE inhibitors)

PARAMETER	OSMOTIC DIURETICS	CARBONIC ANHYDRASE INHIBITORS	THIAZIDE DIURETICS	LOOP DIURETICS	POTASSIUM SPARING DIURETICS
VOLUME	INCREASE	TRANSIENT INCREASE	MODERATE INCREASE	LARGE INCREASE	SMALL INCREASE
SODIUM	NO CHANGE	TRANSIENT INCREASE	MODERATE INCREASE	LARGE INCREASE	SMALL INCREASE
POTASSIUM	NO CHANGE	TRANSIENT INCREASE	MODERATE INCREASE	LARGE INCREASE	MODERATE DECREASE
BICARBONATE	NO CHANGE	TRANSIENT INCREASE	SMALL INCREASE	NO CHANGE	SMALL INCREASE
CHLORIDE	NO CHANGE	TRANSIENT INCREASE	MODERATE INCREASE	LARGE INCREASE	SMALL INCREASE

OVER-THE-COUNTER DRUGS AS DIURETICS

Most over-the-counter drugs promoted as diuretic agents contain caffeine (100 mg) and/or ammonium chloride (about 500 mg). The drugs have, at best, only a mild diuretic action. Caffeine mildly inhibits sodium reabsorption in renal tubules while ammonium chloride metabolism results in urea formation and excretion of a chloride ion. Sodium passively follows the increased chloride load, resulting in mild diuresis.

II.　ANTIDIURETIC DRUGS

A. VASOPRESSIN - Vasopressin (8-arginine vasopressin) is a peptide hormone composed of 9 amino acids. It is synthesized in the hypothalamus, and transported to its site of release in the posterior pituitary. The main stimuli for vasopressin release are hyperosmolality of the blood and volume depletion. (See Posterior Pituitary Hormones in Endocrine Section for Additional Information)

Two types of vasopressin receptors are known. V_1 receptors stimulate contraction of vascular smooth muscles, and V_2 receptors stimulate water reabsorption in the renal tubule through a cyclic AMP dependent mechanism. Vasopressin is found in other areas of the brain, and may promote learning and improve long-term memory.

1. INDICATIONS:

    a. Treatment of diabetes insipidus of pituitary origin
    b. Treatment of bleeding of esophageal varices
    c. Adjunct in hemophilia therapy - increases circulating levels of blood clotting factor VIII.

2. ADVERSE EFFECTS:

    a. Vasoconstriction - may be dangerous in patients with angina
    b. Contraction and cramps of smooth muscles
    c. Water intoxication

3. PREPARATIONS AVAILABLE:

    a. Desmopressin (1-deamino-8-D-arginine vasopressin) nasal spray: A synthetic arginine analog with highest ratio of antidiuretic: vasopressor activities and longest duration of action. Drug of choice.
    b. Lypressin (8-lysine-vasopressin) nasal spray: A synthetic lysine analog
    c. Vasopressin injection - for i.v. use

B. OTHER DRUGS WITH ANTIDIURETIC ACTIVITY

1. CLOFIBRATE: An antilipidemic drug, acts by stimulating vasopressin release from the posterior pituitary

2. CHLORPROPAMIDE: an oral hypoglycemic drug, acts by increasing the action of vasopressin on the renal tubule.

C. VASOPRESSIN ANTAGONISTS

1. DEMECLOCYCLINE

2. LITHIUM CARBONATE

    a. Both demeclocycline and lithium antagonize the renal action of vasopressin, and may be useful in treatment of SIADH (Syndrome of Inappropriate Secretion of Antidiuretic Hormone).

D. TREATMENT OF NEPHROGENIC DIABETES INSIPIDUS

In nephrogenic diabetes insipidus, the kidney is unresponsive to vasopressin, and thiazide diuretics cause a paradoxical reduction in polyuria. The mechanism for this effect is uncertain, but is usually attributed to changes in sodium excretion. Thiazides inhibit NaCl reabsorption in the early segments of the distal tubule, but have little effect in the thick ascending limb, which is involved in concentrating the urine. In the ascending limb, water is reabsorbed along with sodium. Although all thiazides share this effect, **CHLOROTHIAZIDE** is most commonly used to treat this condition.

53

REVIEW QUESTIONS

ONE BEST ANSWER

1. The longest acting peptide analog of antidiuretic hormone is:

   A. Clofibrate
   B. Desmopressin
   C. Enoxaparin
   D. Lypressin
   E. Filagrastim

2. These drugs reduce polyuria in patients who are unresponsive to antidiuretic hormone:

   A. Osmotic diuretics
   B. Vasopressin antagonists
   C. Aldosterone antagonists
   D. Clofibrate and chlorpropamide
   E. Thiazide diuretics

3. The drug useful in SIADH because it antagonizes the renal effects of vasopressin is:

   A. Lypressin
   B Chlorpropamide
   C. Chlorothiazide
   D. Lithium carbonate
   E. Desmopressin

4. The most effective agents for increasing urinary sodium and water excretion:

   A. Inhibit bicarbonate reabsorption in the proximal convoluted tubule
   B. Inhibit chloride ion reabsorption in the ascending loop of Henle
   C. Inhibit sodium reabsorption in the distal convoluted tubule
   D. Inhibit angiotensin converting enzyme activity
   E. Inhibit sodium/potassium exchange in the distal convoluted tubule

5. Potassium retention and hyperkalemia may sometimes be observed with the chronic administration of:

   A. Furosemide
   B. Hydrochlorothiazide
   C. Mannitol
   D. Triamterene
   E. Acetazolamide

6. The urinary excretion of uric acid may be dramatically increased with the administration of:

   A. Furosemide
   B. Chlorthalidone
   C. Acetazolamide
   D. Hydrochlorothiazide
   E. Mannitol

7. Dramatic increases in urinary flow without corresponding increases in urinary sodium excretion are observed with the administration of:

   A. Furosemide
   B. Captopril
   C. Triamterene
   D. Mannitol
   E. Acetazolamide

MATCHING: Each letter can be used more than once or not at all.

From the list below select the letter of the drug most closely associated with the drug action/effect listed below.

A. Aldosterone
B. Triamterene
C. Bretylium
D. Spironolactone
E. Propranolol
F. Disopyramide
G. Flecainide
H. Hydrochlorothiazide

I. Nifedipine
J. Captopril
K. Lidocaine
L. Acetazolamide
M. Mannitol
N. Nitroglycerin
O. Diltiazem

8 Increases urinary bicarbonate ion excretion

9. Directly inhibits sodium-potassium exchange in the distal convoluted tubule

10. Reduces glomerular filtration rate and may precipitate renal failure in patients with impaired renal function

11. Reduces renin release in the kidney

12. Reduces aldosterone release from the adrenal cortex

13. Competitive inhibitor of aldosterone at the aldosterone receptor

14. Reduces the enzymatic formation of angiotensin II from angiotensin I

15. Inhibits carbonic anhydrase

16. Reduces glucose tolerance and may precipitate frank hyperglycemia in some patients

17. Hyperuricemia

18. Metabolic acidosis

CHAPTER 4: DRUGS ACTING ON THE CARDIOVASCULAR SYSTEM

I. CALCIUM ENTRY BLOCKERS

The calcium entry blockers (also termed calcium antagonists, or slow channel blockers) are pharmacologic agents capable of reducing calcium entry through the cell membrane via voltage-dependent, ion specific channels (slow inward current).

Two major channel types exist in cardiac and vascular smooth muscle, the T-type and the L-type channels. The L-type channel is the more physiologically important of the two channels, and is the channel blocked by the compounds termed calcium entry blockers.

Calcium entry blockers differ in their tissue specificity. Drugs such as nifedipine and nicardipine, inhibit calcium entry and smooth muscle contractility with a relative absence of direct effects upon myocardium. The drugs can also prevent or reverse biliary/esophageal spasm.

Diltiazem and verapamil exert significant negative inotropic, chronotropic, and dromotropic effects in the heart in conjunction with smooth muscle relaxation.

All calcium entry blockers :
(1) prevent coronary artery spasm
(2) reduce myocardial O_2 demand

	NIFEDIPINE NICARDIPINE	DILTIAZEM VERAPAMIL
ELECTROPHYSIOLOGY		
SINUS NODE		
DIRECT EFFECT	NONE	*DECREASE*
INDIRECT EFFECT	*INCREASE*	INCREASE
AV NODE		
DIRECT EFFECT	NONE	*DECREASE*
INDIRECT EFFECT	*INCREASE*	INCREASE
HEMODYNAMICS		
PRELOAD	NO CHANGE	NO CHANGE
AFTERLOAD	DECREASE	DECREASE
CONTRACTILITY	NO CHANGE	DECREASE
OXYGEN CONSUMPTION	REDUCED	REDUCED
THERAPEUTIC USEFULNESS		
VARIANT ANGINA	YES	YES
CLASSICAL ANGINA	YES	YES
HYPERTENSION	YES	YES
SUPRAVENTRICULAR TACHYCARDIAS	NO	YES
VENTRICULAR ARRHYTHMIA	NO	NO

ADVERSE EFFECTS

Verapamil - marked negative inotropy; can produce complete AV block if administered in the presence of beta-adrenergic receptor blockade

Diltiazem - modest negative inotropy; can be safely administered in conjunction with beta-adrenergic receptor blockers

<u>Nifedipine, nicardipine</u> - Headache and pedal edema are common, resulting from profound vasodilatation and fluid retention

II. ANTIANGINAL DRUGS

The term **angina**, or **angina pectoris** is used to describe a sudden, temporary substernal pain which often radiates to the left shoulder and/or neck. Anginal pain results from a temporary imbalance between the ability to supply oxygenated blood to cardiac muscle and the oxygen requirements of the tissue. **Acute myocardial ischemia** is the term used to describe the pathophysiologic state wherein the oxygen requirements of the cardiac muscle exceed oxygen delivery via arterial blood. If myocardial ischemia is prolonged, greater than 30 minutes, myocardial cell death will occur. **Unstable angina** is angina at rest and may proceed to myocardial infarction. It is also possible for acute myocardial ischemia to exist in the absence of anginal pain (**silent ischemia**).

The delivery of oxygen to ventricular myocardium is determined by two variables:

(1) oxygen content in arterial blood
(2) myocardial blood flow

Increasing the oxygen content of arterial blood (the hemoglobin is already 95 % saturated at normal inspired oxygen tensions) or increasing oxygen extraction (the heart at rest already extracts more than 90 % of the available oxygen even at rest) are not viable methods for increasing oxygen delivery to working cardiac muscle. Oxygen utilization can only be increased by increased arterial blood flow.

Major factors determining oxygen requirements in cardiac tissue:

(1) **heart rate**
(2) **contractility** - intrinsic force generated by myocardium
(3) **wall tension**
    (a) **preload** - tension exerted on the heart during diastole
    (b) **afterload** - the resistance to blood flow during systole, vascular resistance

INCREASED OXYGEN DEMAND	DECREASED OXYGEN DEMAND
increased heart rate	decreased heart rate
increased heart size	decreased heart size
vasoconstriction	vasodilatation
increased contractility	decreased contractility
exercise, increased sympathetic tone	
hypertension, hypertrophy	
heart failure	

The primary goal in the treatment of angina is <u>not</u> the relief of anginal pain. The primary goal is to restore the balance between oxygen supply and oxygen demand, thereby reversing or preventing myocardial ischemia. Narrowing of the lumen (fixed stenosis) or coronary artery spasm, are frequent complications of coronary atherosclerosis observed in the western world.

Angina produced by a fixed narrowing of a coronary artery lumen (classic angina or exertional angina) and coronary artery spasm (variant angina or Prinzmetal's angina) are distinct clinical entities.

	CORONARY ARTERY SPASM	FIXED, NARROWED LUMEN
ONSET	occurs at rest	occurs with exertion or emotion
VARIATION	unpredictable	day-to-day predictability at fixed exercise level (oxygen demand)
INJURY PATTERN	ST segment elevation (transmural ischemia)	ST segment depression (subendocardial ischemia)
CORONARY LESION	minimal stenosis	fixed lesion > 50% of vessel lumen
TREATMENT	prevent spasm	reduce oxygen demand

A. ORGANIC NITRATES

<u>Nitroglycerin</u> (prototype)
<u>Isosorbide dinitrate, isosorbide mononitrate</u>
<u>Amyl nitrite</u>

Mechanism of Action - Organic nitrates act directly upon vascular smooth muscle to produce arterial and venous dilation. By reducing preload and afterload, **myocardial oxygen consumption is reduced**. In the presence of a fixed stenosis, coronary blood flow is not altered. The decrease in mean blood pressure produces reflex activation of the sympathetic nervous system. Increases in heart rate and contractility **partially reverse** the decrease in oxygen consumption produced by arterial and venous vasodilation, and can be blocked by beta-adrenergic receptor antagonists. In patients with variant angina, the organic nitrates can prevent or reverse coronary artery spasm. **Organic nitrates are effective for the treatment of both effort-induced angina and coronary artery spasm.**

Absorption, Fate, and Excretion - The organic nitrates are rapidly and extensively metabolized by the liver. Except for isosorbide mononitrate (which has good oral bioavailability and efficacy), only a small fraction of an orally administered dose appears unchanged in the peripheral blood. The drugs are lipid-soluble and are well-absorbed through the skin and mucous membranes.

Mode of Administration

Oral - Only isosorbide mononitrate is effective with oral administration

Sublingual Tablets - Nitroglycerin and isosorbide are rapidly absorbed through the oral mucosa. Therapeutic effects are observed within 2-4 mins, but last for only 1 - 2 hrs.

Transdermal Administration - Well-absorbed through skin from ointments and sustained release patches. The therapeutic effects of the ointment persist for 4 - 8 hrs and the sustained release preparation can maintain stable blood levels of nitroglycerin for 24 hrs. Usefulness limited by rapid tolerance development.

Intravenous Nitroglycerin- IV infusion. Used in the treatment of myocardial infarction.

Inhalation - Amyl nitrite is volatile and is administered by inhalation.

Adverse Effects

Headache - tolerance develops with repeated use
Postural hypotension

Tolerance - The continued, uninterrupted use of organic nitrates results in tolerance. Subsequent doses of nitrates produce little hemodynamic response. The use of dermal nitrates should not extend for more than 12 - 16 hrs of any 24 hr period and must include a nitrate-free interval between doses.

B. CALCIUM ENTRY BLOCKERS - see the calcium entry blockers section

C. B-ADRENERGIC RECEPTOR ANTAGONISTS

Propranolol (prototype)

B-adrenergic receptor antagonists **reduce myocardial oxygen consumption.** The reduction in myocardial oxygen consumption results from both a decrease in resting heart rate and a decrease in myocardial contractility. The decreased oxygen consumption is partially negated by small increases in preload and afterload. **The B-adrenergic receptor antagonists are useful for the prophylaxis of effort-induced angina, but are not effective for the acute termination of effort-induced angina or for the treatment of coronary artery spasm.**

B-adrenergic receptor antagonists are used in combination with organic nitrates. The drugs antagonize the increased sympathetic nervous system activity observed with the organic nitrates.

	NITRATES	BETA-BLOCKERS
HEART RATE	SMALL INCREASE	LARGE DECREASE
CONTRACTILITY	SMALL INCREASE	LARGE DECREASE
PRELOAD	LARGE DECREASE	SMALL INCREASE
AFTERLOAD	SMALL DECREASE	SMALL INCREASE
OXYGEN CONSUMPTION	MODERATE DECREASE	MODERATE DECREASE

*note that the hemodynamic actions of the nitrates compliment those of the beta-blockers and are the basis for their concomitant use in the therapy of effort-induced angina

III. ANTIARRHYTHMIC DRUGS

A. CARDIAC ACTION POTENTIAL

phase 0: rapid depolarization due to rapid sodium entry

the maximum rate of voltage change during phase 0 (dV/dt) determines conduction velocity

phase 1: rapid, initial outward movement of potassium ions (transient outward current)
present in rapid response tissues only (absent in slow response tissues)

phase 2: sustained calcium entry (L-type calcium current)

calcium entry during phase two is necessary for cardiac muscle contraction

phase 3: outward potassium ion movement (outward current) returns membrane to resting potential

phase 4: spontaneous depolarization

a mixture of inward currents and reduced outward potassium currents producing spontaneous depolarization

The velocity of conduction in ventricular tissue determines the duration of the QRS interval in the surface electrocardiogram (EKG). The duration of the action potential in ventricular muscle determines the duration of the QT interval in the surface electrocardiogram (EKG).

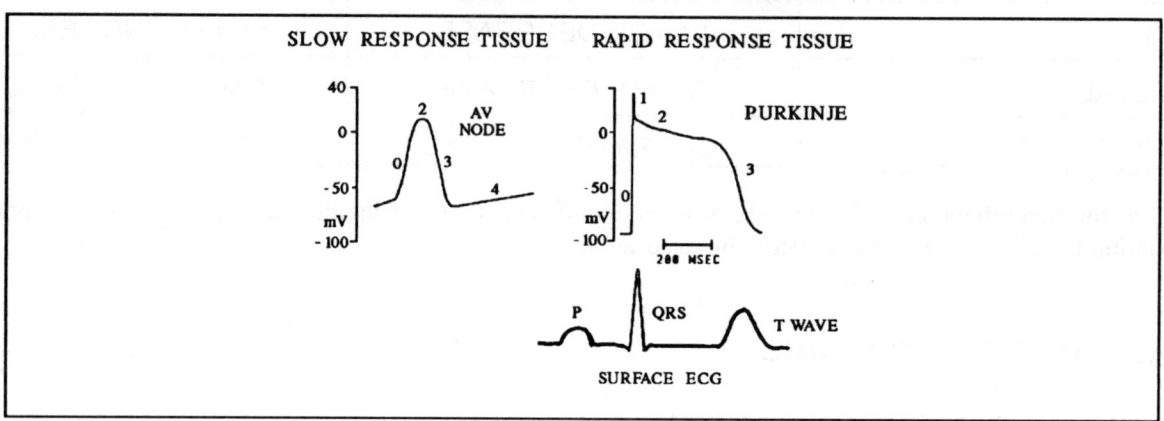

The heart contains two types of tissues with distinct electrical properties. Slow response and fast response tissues respond differently to antiarrhythmic drugs.

PARAMETER	SLOW RESPONSE TISSUE	FAST RESPONSE TISSUE
RESTING POTENTIAL	-65 to -30 mV	-95 to -65 mV
PHASE 0 UPSTROKE	2 to 20 V/sec	100 to 800 V/sec
ACTION POTENTIAL AMPLITUDE	70 to 70 mV	80 to 120 mV
ACTION POTENTIAL DURATION	75 to 150 msec	150 to 600 msec
INWARD CURRENT	I_{na} (sodium) and $I_{Ca(L)}$ (calcium)	I_{na} (sodium)
CONDUCTION VELOCITY	0.01 to 0.1 M/sec	0.3 to 2 M/sec
REFRACTORINESS	250 to 500 msec, post-repolarization	150 to 400 msec
TISSUES	SA node, AV node	atrium, ventricle

B. CLASSIFICATION OF CARDIAC ARRHYTHMIAS

1. **Atrial Flutter** - The atrial rhythm is both **rapid and regular** (300 - 400 /minute). One of every two (2:1 block) or three atrial beats (3:1 block) is conducted to the ventricle through the AV node. The ventricular heart rate (133 - 200 /minute) is regular, but is too rapid to allow optimal ventricular filling during diastole. Cardiac output and exercise tolerance are reduced. The goal of therapy is to slow the ventricular heart rate. This can be accomplished by:

a. Converting atrial flutter to atrial fibrillation
b. Decreasing the ability of the AV node to conduct atrial impulses to the ventricles

2. **Atrial Fibrillation** - The atrial rhythm is **rapid** (400 - 600 /minute) and **irregular**. The ventricular rate is also rapid and irregular (100 - 150 /minute). The ventricular rate is slower than observed with atrial flutter, but both cardiac output and exercise tolerance are reduced. The electrical properties of the AV node (slow response tissue) are such that as the atrial rate increases over 200 /minute, conduction through the AV node is slower and more likely to block. Therapy is directed to

   a. convert atrial fibrillation to sinus rhythm (electrical cardioversion), or
   b. decreasing the ability of the AV node to conduct atrial impulses to the ventricle impulses from exciting the ventricles.

   Class I antiarrhythmic drug therapy may also be used to suppress the recurrence of atrial fibrillation/flutter.

3. **Ventricular Premature Beats** - Premature ventricular beats are ventricular beats originating in the ventricles. The premature beats usually do not reduce cardiac output. Many patients with frequent premature ventricular beats may be bothered by palpitations. The goal of therapy is to reduce the number of ventricular premature beats and improve patient comfort.

4. **Ventricular Tachycardia and Ventricular Fibrillation** - Ventricular tachycardia (200 - 400 beats/min) and ventricular fibrillation (>400 beats/min) are rapid rhythms originating in the ventricle. Ventricular tachycardia can be self-terminating or sustained (lasting for more than 30 sec). Ventricular fibrillation is invariably fatal unless electrical defibrillation is performed. Patients with ventricular tachycardia and heart disease have a high probability of developing ventricular fibrillation. Ventricular tachycardia leading to ventricular fibrillation is the leading cause of death in the United States. The goal of drug therapy is to prevent the recurrence of ventricular tachycardia and fibrillation and prolong life.

C. CLASS I ANTIARRHYTHMIC DRUGS

Class IA -	Quinidine Procainamide Disopyramide	prolong action potential duration/QT interval slow conduction/prolong QRS interval at moderate and fast heart rates
Class IB -	Lidocaine Mexiletine Tocainide	shorten action potential duration/QT interval slow conduction/prolong QRS interval only at fast heart rates

Class IC -   Propafenone   no prominent effect upon action potential duration
             Flecainide   slow conduction/prolong QRS interval at slow,
             Moricizine   moderate, and fast heart rates

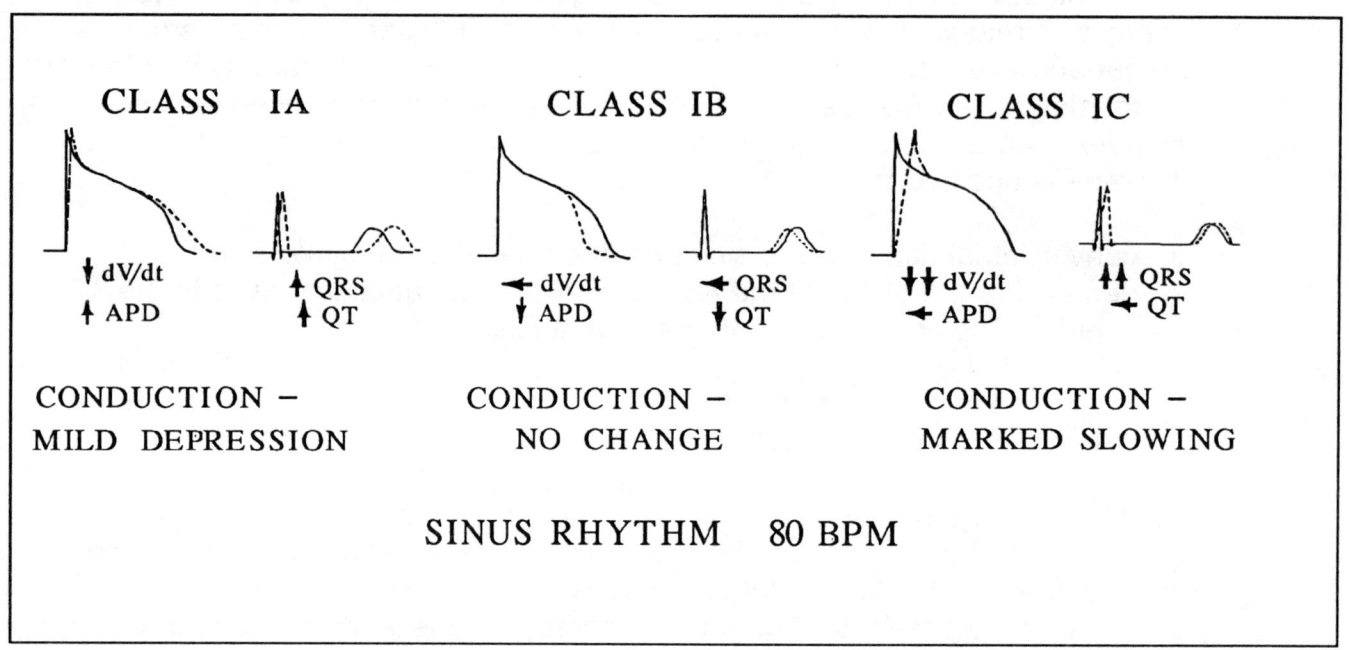

All Class I antiarrhythmic agents slow conduction in atrial and ventricular tissue. All are local anesthetics. Their actions on the AV node are different for the individual agents.

Class I antiarrhythmic drugs may cause life-threatening arrhythmias (ventricular tachycardia or ventricular fibrillation) in patients treated for less serious arrhythmias. One life-threatening ventricular arrhythmia produced by both Class IA and Class III agents is torsades de pointes.

1. QUINIDINE, PROCAINAMIDE, AND DISOPYRAMIDE

All Class IA drugs have <u>anticholinergic</u> actions. The drugs (1) improve AV nodal conduction by antagonizing the actions of the vagus nerve upon the AV node and (2) directly depress AV nodal conduction. The net effect upon AV nodal conduction is variable. <u>The drugs should not be used alone for the treatment of atrial flutter or atrial fibrillation as the ventricular heart rate may dramatically increase and cardiac output decrease.</u> All three drugs depress myocardial contractility and can worsen existing heart failure.

Adverse Effects

    dry eyes, dry mouth, urinary retention - <u>anticholinergic</u>
    heart failure - all are negative inotropic agents
    worsening of arrhythmia - torsades de pointes

    cinchonism - quinidine only (quinidine is d-isomer of quinine)
       ringing in ears
    diarrhea - 30% incidence with quinidine

    acute lupus erythematosus - procainamide only
       skin rash, muscle weakness, arthralgia - joint pain

2. LIDOCAINE, TOCAINIDE, and MEXILETINE

Class 1B drugs have little effect upon AV nodal conduction or myocardial contractility. Lidocaine is rapidly metabolized in the liver. Lidocaine has a short-plasma half-life and is used as an IV infusion only in a hospital setting. Tocainide and mexiletine are used orally for long-term therapy.

Adverse Effects

    central nervous system - act as local anesthetics in brain
       sedation - low doses
       muscle twitching, vertigo - moderate dosages
       convulsions - higher doses

    agranulocytosis - dangerous but uncommon side effect seen with tocainide

3. FLECAINIDE, PROPAFENONE, and MORICIZINE

Flecainide, propafenone, and moricizine slow conduction in <u>all</u> cardiac tissues (including AV node) and also depresses cardiac contractility.

Adverse Effects

    heart failure - all Class IC drugs are negative inotropic agents
    worsening of cardiac arrhythmias - the drugs may increase mortality when administered to patients surviving myocardial infarction
    headache

D. CLASS II ANTIARRHYTHMIC DRUGS

B-adrenergic receptor antagonists

Class II agents are used :

1. to depress AV nodal conduction with atrial flutter/fibrillation
2. to prevent ventricular fibrillation during the first 2 years following myocardial infarction.

Propranolol is a beta-adrenergic receptor antagonist which is also a local anesthetic and hence is also a Class I antiarrhythmic drugs.

The pharmacology of the beta-adrenergic receptor antagonists is discussed under adrenergic drugs.

E. CLASS III ANTIARRHYTHMIC DRUGS

Amiodarone
Bretylium
Sotalol

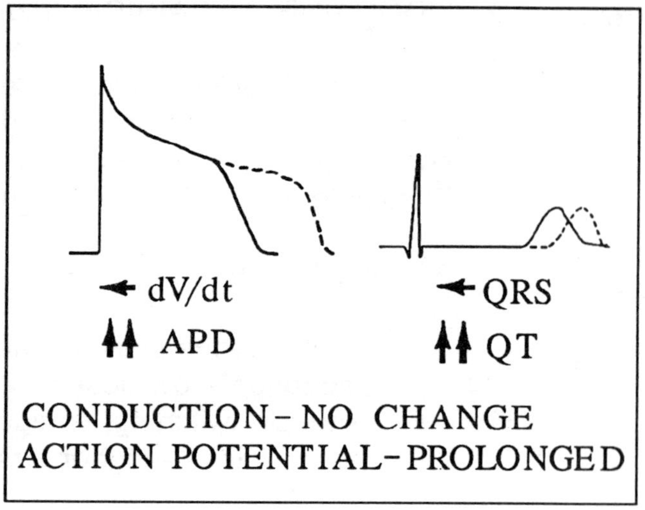

The Class III antiarrhythmic drugs prolong action potential duration without slowing conduction velocity. Bretylium, amiodarone, and sotalol are used for the treatment of recurrent ventricular tachycardia/fibrillation. Because of the high incidence of serious side effects, the Class III drugs are restricted for severe, life-threatening arrhythmias. Bretylium is used only in an acute hospital setting and is administered parenterally.

The half-life of amiodarone in man is approximately 30 days. There is a prolonged time to achieve efficacy with oral administration and drug effects are prolonged after drug withdrawal.

Adverse Effects:

Amiodarone: corneal opacities
photosensitivity - gray-blue skin rash
thyroid dysfunction - drug contains iodine atoms
peripheral neuropathy
life-threatening pulmonary toxicity - uncommon, but may not remit with drug withdrawal

Bretylium: hypertension followed by hypotension - the drug initially releases norepinephrine from sympathetic nerve endings followed by an inhibition of sympathetic neuronal release of norepinephrine with nerve firing

Sotalol: B-blocker, torsades de pointes

F. CLASS IV ANTIARRHYTHMIC AGENTS

Calcium entry blockers: <u>Verapamil</u>
<u>Diltiazem</u>

Class IV drugs inhibit calcium entry through L-type calcium channels in myocardium.

The calcium entry blockers are used for (1) for the treatment of atrial flutter/fibrillation and (2) for acute termination of AV nodal reentry

Verapamil and diltiazem depress AV nodal transmission. Nifedipine and nicardipine, although excellent vasodilators and antianginal drugs, are poor inhibitors of AV nodal transmission and are ineffective as antiarrhythmic drugs.

Verapamil administration may produce sinus arrest or complete AV nodal blockade in the presence of beta-adrenergic receptor blockade.

The hemodynamic effects and adverse effects of the calcium entry blockers are discussed in the calcium antagonists section.

B. ADENOSINE

Adenosine is an effective drug for the acute termination of AV node reentry. Adenosine (1) increases vagal tone to the AV node and (2) may directly depress AV nodal conduction.

The drug is administered as an IV bolus (just as fast as you can inject it) and has a plasma half-life of a few seconds (taken up by red blood cells). A repeat bolus can be given again within minutes if the first dose is ineffective. Adverse effects are limited to (1) transient dyspnea and (2) flushing.

IV.   THERAPY OF CONGESTIVE HEART FAILURE

Digitalis glycosides have been the mainstay of therapy for chronic congestive heart failure (CHF) for centuries. Recently, however, the effectiveness of digitalis glycosides has been questioned in relation to their effect on long term survival benefits. Present therapeutic approaches to the treatment of CHF require a thorough understanding of the pathophysiology of CHF because a) the long term treatment of CHF with digitalis is purely symptomatic, b) significant toxicity occurs in about 10% or more of patients receiving the drug, and c) only about 25% of chronic CHF patients with a normal sinus rhythm are benefitted.

Pathophysiology

Congestive heart failure (CHF) is a pathophysiologic state in which cardiac output is inadequate to meet the demands of metabolizing tissue. The mismatch between cardiac output and demand may result from either a basic cardiac dysfunction with low cardiac output and normal peripheral requirements (low output failure) or from increased tissue demands beyond those which can be met by a normal or high but inadequate cardiac output (high output failure). Congestive heart failure is an extremely complex condition in which a variety of primary pathologic events are blended with varying compensatory mechanisms to produce the commonly recognized spectrum of clinical symptoms and signs.

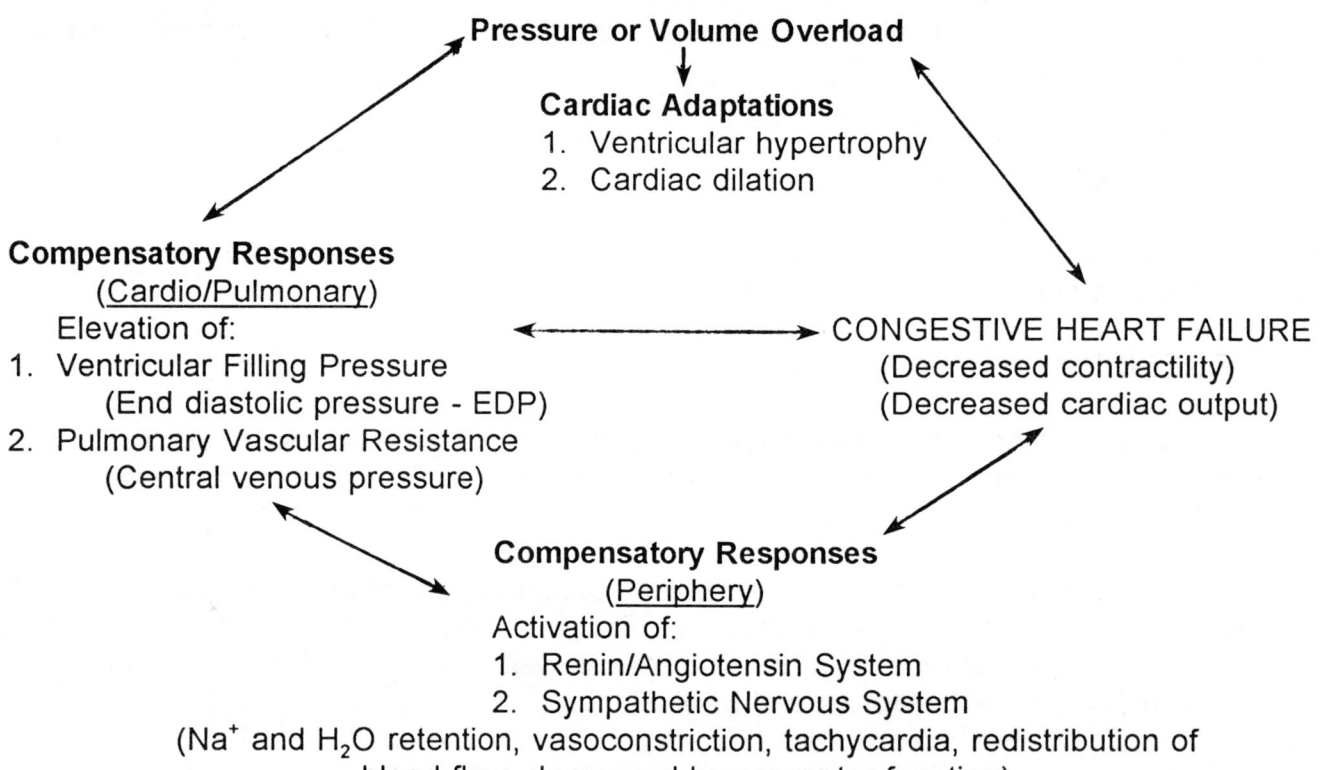

(Hypertension, valvular disease, myocardial infarct, cardiomyopathy)

Pressure or Volume Overload

Cardiac Adaptations
1. Ventricular hypertrophy
2. Cardiac dilation

Compensatory Responses
(Cardio/Pulmonary)
Elevation of:
1. Ventricular Filling Pressure
   (End diastolic pressure - EDP)
2. Pulmonary Vascular Resistance
   (Central venous pressure)

CONGESTIVE HEART FAILURE
(Decreased contractility)
(Decreased cardiac output)

Compensatory Responses
(Periphery)
Activation of:
1. Renin/Angiotensin System
2. Sympathetic Nervous System
(Na$^+$ and H$_2$O retention, vasoconstriction, tachycardia, redistribution of blood flow, decreased baroreceptor function)

Because of our vastly improved understanding of the pathophysiology of CHF, the last decade has ushered in a new era in the management of CHF. The older mainstays of treatment (digitalis, sodium restriction and diuretics) in many instances have been augmented or supplanted by the use of a diverse group of drugs generally referred to as vasodilators. Clinical studies have shown that the survival rate in patients with severe CHF treated with vasodilators is prolonged. Although attempts have been made to categorize these drugs as "agents for preload reduction" or "agents for afterload reduction", most vasodilators have direct and/or indirect effects on both the arterial and venous beds, thus reducing both preload and afterload.

Despite setbacks in developing other new therapies for CHF, the angiotensin converting enzyme (ACE) inhibitors are gaining acceptance as important therapeutic options.

Drug Management of CHF

In CHF the depressed contractile performance of the myocardium is aggravated by increases in preload and afterload related in part to arterial and venous constriction. Vasodilator drugs exert their salutary effect on left ventricular performance by decreasing aortic impedance and/or increasing venous capacitance. This results in an increased stroke volume and a decreased filling pressure.

A. DIURETICS

Diuretics promote the excretion of sodium and water. By reducing the elevated circulating blood volume in CHF, diuretics may reduce the preload and edema. Some also may have a vasodilator action. Treatment of CHF may include salt restriction and diuretics, however, recent studies indicate that diuretics alone are inadequate, although they may provide some symptomatic relief. Diuretics should be used in conjunction with a vasodilator or digoxin.

B. VASODILATORS

1. DIRECT SMOOTH MUSCLE RELAXANTS

a. Nitroglycerin is used for short-term intravenous treatment of severe CHF. It dilates large capacitance veins and reduces preload. Development of tolerance limits its therapeutic usefulness.

b. Nitroprusside is a potent relaxant for both veins and arteries. It use is limited to short-term intravenous therapy. Its short half-life allows for titration and makes it beneficial in acute or severe refractory CHF.

c. Hydralazine is primarily an arteriolar vasodilator and may be beneficial in reducing afterload in CHF. Tolerance may develop to this drug and it also may worsen fluid retention.

2. BLOCKING AGENTS

Prazosin selectively blocks postsynaptic $alpha_1$-adrenergic receptors and reduces afterload by relaxing arteriolar and venous smooth muscle. Cardiac output increases with relatively little or no reflex tachycardia. Prazosin also may have some CNS sympatho-inhibitory action.

3. ENZYME INHIBITORS

Angiotensin converting enzyme (ACE) inhibitors, along with digitalis and diuretics, are now considered as first-line drugs for therapy of CHF.

a. Captopril acutely decreases systemic vascular resistance, venous tone and mean blood pressure while producing a sustained increase in cardiac output. Recent clinical studies have reported symptomatic improvement and reduced mortality in patients with CHF. Exercise tolerance in patients with refractory CHF is improved and salt and water retention is reduced. Adverse effects include hyperkalemia, first-dose hypertension, taste disturbances, and rash; some patients develop a persistent cough. Captopril is moderately well absorbed after oral administration.

b. Enalapril has a longer duration of action than captopril and can be given less frequently, once or twice daily. It is considered a pro-drug which is metabolized to an active metabolite, enalaprilat. Adverse effects are similar to those for captopril.

c. Lisinopril is one of several new ACE inhibitors and can be given once daily.

C. INOTROPIC AGENTS

Although positive inotropic agents act by several mechanisms to increase cardiac muscle contractility, the ultimate final common denominator for the inotropic action is the increased concentration of intracytoplasmic calcium in myocardial cells. In the failing heart, inotropic agents shift the Frank-Starling curve towards a more normal position. This results in a decrease of stroke work, a reduction in myocardial oxygen consumption and an improvement in cardiac output.

1. DIGITALIS GLYCOSIDES

The most clinically important glycosides, digoxin and digitoxin, come from *Digitalis sp.* plants (foxglove). The active principles (aglycones) are steroid structures; binding characteristics are affected by their attachment to sugars.

All of the therapeutically useful and toxic effects of digitalis are thought to be attributable to inhibition of Na^+/K^+-ATPase (the digitalis receptor) located on the outside of the myocardial cell membrane. Normally, this Na^+/K^+ "pump" is responsible for the exchange of these ions across the membrane; when the pump is inhibited, Na^+ accumulates intracellularly. Secondarily, the decreased Na^+ gradient affects Na^+/Ca^{++} exchange and Ca^{++} accumulates inside the cell.. Consequently, more intracytoplasmic Ca^{++} (stored in the sarcoplasmic reticulum) is available for release and interaction with the contractile proteins during the excitation-contraction coupling process. Thus, with therapeutic doses, their is an increase in the contractile force generated. Toxicity to digitalis also relates to inhibition of the receptor (Na^+/K^+-ATPase). Inhibition of the Na^+/K^+ pump affects the K^+ gradient and this may lead to a significant reduction of intracellular K^+, predisposing the heart towards arrhythmias. Likewise Ca^{++} overload also may contribute to serious arrhythmias as well. Thus, there is a narrow margin (low therapeutic index) between those doses of digitalis that improve myocardial mechanics and hemodynamics and those doses that cause electrophysiological effects which are arrhythmogenic.

Cardiovascular Actions of Digitalis:

The fundamental action of digitalis is to increase the force and velocity of cardiac contraction (increases rate of development of tension in the myocardium - dT/dt). There is a direct positive inotropic action on the myocardium of both nonfailing and failing hearts; however, the hemodynamic consequences of this action may be quite different because of the compensatory mechanisms that are activated during the state of failure. There is a marked increase in cardiac output in the failing heart but little to no effect on cardiac output in the nonfailing heart as baroreceptor reflexes remain fully active (inotropic action offset by autonomic nervous system effects).

The second most important action of digitalis is to slow the heart rate. The magnitude of slowing is dependent upon pre-existing vagal or sympathetic tone. Both direct and indirect actions, mediated by the vagus nerve, contribute to the decrease in heart rate. These are:

a. Slowing the discharge rate of the normal pacemaker, the sino-atrial (S-A) node.
b. Slowing conduction through the atrio-ventricular (A-V) node; prolonging the refractory period of the A-V nodal cells.

Other direct effects, however, may be antagonized by an opposing vagal effect; i.e., atrial muscle refractory period is shortened - an indirect predominately vagal effect.

When normal ionic exchanges across cell membranes are inhibited by digitalis, complex, dose-dependent electrophysiological effects are observed. As therapeutic concentrations are exceeded, the automaticity of secondary latent, ectopic pacemaker cells is increased. This most likely results from Ca^{++} overload which can cause oscillatory afterdepolarizations to occur after an action potential. Premature ventricular contractions, ventricular tachycardia and ventricular fibrillation are serious arrhythmias that occur in digitalis toxic patients and they are thought to be triggered by afterdepolarizations that reach the threshold potential. Characteristic electrocardiographic changes produced by digitalis may herald impending toxicity. They are: P-R interval prolongation (due to slowed conduction through the A-V node), S-T segment depression, T wave inversion and Q-T interval shortening.

Digitalis acts not only on cardiac muscle but also on smooth muscle. It acts on the digitalis receptor in smooth muscle to increase intracellular Ca^{++}.

Vascular Smooth Muscle: Digitalis directly constricts arterial and venous smooth muscle. When no failure exists, peripheral vascular resistance increases and blood pressure may increase. In heart failure, with a marked compensatory increase in sympathetic tone, no additional constrictor effect occurs. Instead, there is an apparent <u>vasodilation</u> and <u>peripheral</u> vascular <u>resistance falls</u> as an <u>indirect</u> <u>consequence</u> of <u>improved output</u> and <u>hemodynamic status</u>.

<u>Autonomic Nervous System</u>: Digitalis directly stimulates the Xth (vagal) nucleus in the brain. The parasympathetic nervous system actions of digitalis correlate with its therapeutic effects (vagally - mediated slowing of heart rate, inhibition at A-V node, etc.). The sympathetic stimulation also occurring with digitalis may facilitate the development of toxicity and arrhythmias.

TO SUMMARIZE: In CHF patients digitalis glycosides can exert the following effects by direct and/or indirect actions: increase myocardial contractility, slow heart rate, decrease end diastolic pressure and volume, increase stroke output and cardiac output, and decrease stroke work. When excessive sympathetic tone and neurohumoral substances gradually are withdrawn as hemodynamics improve, blood volume is reduced, congestion improves, heart size returns towards normal, oxygen consumption decreases, and mechanical efficiency of the heart improves.

<u>Adverse Effects</u>: Gastrointestinal effects are common and are among the earliest signs of toxicity; anorexia, nausea, vomiting and abdominal pain occur. Digitalis causes direct chemical stimulation of the chemoreceptor emetic trigger zone in the area postrema (floor of 4th ventricle) leading to nausea and vomiting. Neuralgic pain (simulating trigeminal neuralgia), fatigue, headache, and drowsiness also are considered early signs of toxicity. More serious signs are: disorientation, delirium, personality changes, visual disturbances (photophobia, halos, yellow vision), and rarely hallucinations or convulsions. Even more rarely, gynecomastia, galactorrhea or hypersensitivity reactions may occur. Digitalis toxicity is exacerbated most commonly by K^+ depletion (with diuretics) but also by sympathomimetic agents, Ca^{++}, Mg^{++}, hypoxia, and an increased heart rate.

Digitalis preparations differ in onset and duration of action (lipid/water solubility). All have the same therapeutic index, actions and toxicities. Consider them as <u>dangerous drugs</u>. To treat toxicity, discontinue the drug, correct potassium deficiency and use digoxin antibodies (Fab fragments).

<u>DIGOXIN</u>	<u>DIGITOXIN</u>
More water soluble	More lipid soluble
Can give orally or i.v.	Usually given orally
Well absorbed (up to 75%)	Completely absorbed (100%)
Onset of action - fast	Onset of action - slow
Half-life about 1.5 days	Half-life five to seven days
Primarily excreted by kidney	Extensively metabolized by liver

2. PHOSPHODIESTERASE (PDE) INHIBITORS

    a. <u>Amrinone</u>: By inhibiting PDE, this drug increases cAMP and causes an increase in intracellular calcium levels. It is a positive inotropic agent with vasodilator activity, as well. It is used infrequently and only then is given parenterally for short-term management of CHF patients refractory to digitalis, preload or afterload reduction. It has considerable toxicity and has proved unacceptable for long term use. Adverse effects include fever, nausea, vomiting, hypersensitivity reactions, hepatotoxicity, and thrombocytopenia.

    b. <u>Milrinone</u> is a congener of amrinone and probably acts by a similar mechanism on PDE. It has similar adverse effects but is better tolerated.

3. BETA-ADRENERGIC RECEPTOR AGONISTS

Drugs in this class stimulate cardiac <u>beta</u>$_1$-adrenergic receptors by activation of adenylate cyclase. They rarely are used in heart failure because they increase heart rate, may cause arrhythmias and increase oxygen consumption. Their role in the treatment of chronic CHF remains to be demonstrated.

    a. <u>Dopamine</u> at low doses increases myocardial contractility. It must be given by i.v. infusion. It may be useful in acute severe failure for its positive inotropic action. Its action in the kidney on dopamine receptors increases renal blood flow.

    b. <u>Dobutamine</u> stimulates <u>alpha</u>$_1$- and <u>beta</u>-receptors in both heart and blood vessels but selectively stimulates the cardiac <u>beta</u>$_1$-receptors to produce its inotropic action. It must be given by i.v. infusion.

V. THERAPY OF HYPERLIPOPROTEINEMIAS

A. CLOFIBRATE
    1. Lowers VLDL and plasma triglycerides, probably by stimulating lipoprotein lipase. Lowers cholesterol by inhibiting its synthesis and enhancing excretion in the bile.
    2. Used for both hypertriglyceridemia and hypercholesterolemia.
    3. Contraindicated in pregnancy or patients with impaired renal or hepatic function.
    4. It displaces acidic drugs (e.g., warfarin, phenytoin) from plasma proteins, thus a reduced dose of anticoagulant (or other drug) is required.
    5. Adverse effects: GI disturbances, muscle weakness, rash. Its long term use may increase the incidence of thromboembolism, angina, arrhythmias, gallstones.

B. CHOLESTYRAMINE AND CHOLESTIPOL
1. Lower LDL and plasma cholesterol. Drugs of choice for hypercholesterolemia.
2. Insoluble steroid binding (ion-exchange) resins that are not absorbed but which bind bile acids in gut, preventing their absorption. They increase the hepatic conversion of cholesterol to bile acids, thereby reducing the cholesterol available through the enterohepatic circulation for production of plasma lipids.
3. Adverse effects: Unpleasant taste and smell, nausea, constipation, steatorrhea, deficiency of fat-soluble vitamins (e.g., vitamin K). Compliance may be a problem..
4. May interfere with the absorption of other drugs given concurrently (e.g., warfarin).

C. NICOTINIC ACID (NIACIN)
1. Lowers both cholesterol and triglycerides.
2. It inhibits triglyceride lipase activation by lipolytic hormones and also reduces LDL synthesis.
3. Adverse effects: Cutaneous flushing, burning and itching are common, as is GI irritation, nausea and vomiting. Activation of peptic ulcer, abnormally high liver enzyme levels, hyperglycemia, and hyperuricemia occur infrequently.
* Nicotinamide is not effective in lowering lipids although it acts interchangeably with nicotinic acid as a vitamin.

D. GEMFIBROZIL
1. Similar to clofibrate, but more commonly causes skin rash.
2. Lowers VLDL and triglycerides by activating lipoprotein lipase; HDL may increase.

E. PROBUCOL
1. Decreases LDL and cholesterol by an unknown mechanism but HDL also may be lowered. Used for hypercholesterolemia if other drugs ineffective.
2. Side effects include diarrhea, flatulence, nausea, abdominal pain

F. LOVASTATIN (Simvastatin, Pravastatin)
1. Competitively inhibit HMG-CoA reductase, rate limiting enzyme in cholesterol synthesis, and cause significant reductions in LDL; HDL may be elevated.
2. Adverse effects to this new class of drugs appear minimal to date; myositis, lens opacities and increased liver enzymes in plasma have been reported.

VI.   ANTIHYPERTENSIVE THERAPY

1. Clearly reduces cerebrovascular disease, heart failure, renal insufficiency and possibly the risk of myocardial infarction.
2. Is indicated whenever:
   a. target organs are affected;
   b. minimally elevated blood pressure is associated with other cardiovascular risk factors; e.g., smoking, diabetes, obesity, hyperlipidemia and genetic predisposition;
   c. persistent blood pressure elevations above 145/90 or 170-180/95 in the elderly.
3. May initially consist of reducing salt intake and weight, and modification of other risk factors.

A. HYPOTENSIVE DIURETICS

1. SULFONAMIDE DIURETICS (THIAZIDES, CHLOROTHIAZIDE, HYDROCHLOROTHIAZIDE):

   a. Orally effective - useful for mild to moderate hypertension; standard now in therapy of hypertension; frequently given along with other antihypertensive medication and can potentiate the action of other antihypertensive drugs.
   b. Precise mode of action poorly understood; antihypertensive effects during the first few weeks of treatment have been related to decreased circulating blood volume and decreased cardiac output, but these return to nearly normal values after a few weeks; action may in part be related to a depletion or redistribution of sodium; may act by direct arteriolar dilation.
   c. Antihypertensive actions of all thiazides are comparable.
   d. K^+ loss leads to hypokalemic alkalosis; rarely a problem in normal patients; may be problematic in patients with cardiac arrhythmias, especially if on digitalis or those with severe liver disease.
   e. Some increase in plasma lipid concentrations.

ANTI-HYPERTENSIVE DRUGS

Mechanism of Action		Drug Category	Drugs
Diuretics	A)	Thiazides and related agents	Hydrochlorothiazide (Hydrodiuril) Chlorthalidone (Hygroton)
	B)	Loop diuretics	Furosemide (Lasix) Ethacrynic acid (Edecrin) Bumethanide (Bumex)
	C)	Potassium-sparing diuretics	Spironolactone (Aldactone) Triamterine (Dyrenium) Amiloride (Midamor)
Sympatholytic Drugs	A)	Centrally acting agents	Clonidine (Catapres) Methyldopa (Aldomet)
	B)	Beta-adrenoceptor antagonists	Propranolol (Inderal) Metaprolol (Lopressor) Nadolol (Corgard) Atenolol (Tenormin) Pindolol (Visken) Timolol (Blocadren)
	C)	Alpha-adrenoceptor antagonists	Prazosin (Minipress)
	D)	Mixed antagonist	Labetalol (Normodyne, Trandate, Vescal)
	E)	Adrenergic neuron blocking agents	Reserpine (Serpasil) Guanethidine (Ismelin)
	F)	Ganglionic blockade	Trimethaphan (Arfonad)
Direct Vasodilators	A)	Arterial vasodilators	Hydralazine (Apresoline) Minoxidil (Ioniten) Diazoxide (Hyperstat)
	B)	Calcium antagonists	Nifedipine (Procardia) Diltiazem (Cardizem)
	C)	Arterial and venous vasodilators	Sodium nitroprusside (Nipride, Nitropress)
Angiotensin Antagonists	A)	Converting enzyme inhibitors	Captopril (Capoten) Enalapril (Vasotec) Lisinopril (Prinivil, Zestril)

2. LOOP DIURETICS (FUROSEMIDE, ETHACRYNIC ACID, BUMETHANIDE):

   a. More potent with more potential for side effects; increased renin; hypokalemia; hyperglycemia; hyperuricemia
   b. Thiazides more effective than loop diuretics in patients without edema.

3. POTASSIUM-SPARING DIURETICS:

   a. Spironolactone: As effective as thiazides but more side effects. May be useful in patients with hyperuricemia, hypokalemia, glucose intolerance. A drug of choice in patients with primary aldosteronism. Competitive antagonist to aldosterone.

b. <u>Triamterene and Amiloride</u>: May be given along with the thiazide to prevent potassium depletion (have little hypotensive action alone).

B. SYMPATHOLYTIC DRUGS

1. CNS SYMPATHO-INHIBITORY DRUGS:

a. <u>Clonidine</u>:
1) CNS stimulation of <u>alpha$_2$</u>-adrenoceptors causes inhibition of sympathetic tone. Effects antagonized by yohimbine; long acting.
2) Very lipophylic; orally administered; may be given with transdermal patch.
3) Side effects include xerostomia (dry mouth); sedation; fluid retention (use with diuretic).
4) Withdrawal may precipitate hypertensive crisis; may be treated with labetalol, <u>beta</u> antagonist.

b. <u>Methyldopa</u>:
Metabolized to <u>alpha</u>-methyl norepinephrine (<u>alpha</u>-MNE) which can displace and deplete NE in storage sites; research indicates that the antihypertensive effect is by CNS action; causes drowsiness and depression; may act on CNS <u>alpha</u>-2 receptors to decrease sympathetic tone by <u>alpha</u>-MNE (also indirect decrease of renin release).

2. BETA-ADRENERGIC RECEPTOR BLOCKING AGENTS: (see Chapter 2)

a. <u>Propranolol</u>:
1) Non-selective <u>beta$_1$</u> and <u>beta$_2$</u> blocker.
2) Mechanism of action: decreases cardiac output; decreases sympathetic tone <u>via</u> central action and decrease renin release.
3) Adverse effects: bradycardia, congestive heart failure, mental depression and bronchospasm.

b. <u>Nadolol</u>:
1) Non-selective <u>beta$_1$</u> and <u>beta$_2$</u> blocker but lacks direct myocardial depressant effect as propranolol.
2) Long duration of action; can be used once a day.
3) Mechanism of action: similar to propranolol.
4) Adverse effects: bradycardia, dizziness, bronchospasm and cardiac failure.

c. <u>Metoprolol and Atenolol</u>:
1) More selective <u>beta$_1$</u> blocker (cardiac selective).
2) Mechanism of action: similar to propranolol.
3) Adverse effects: headache, insomnia, dizziness.
4) Precaution: could be used in asthmatics for treatment of hypertension but requires caution.

d. Pindolol:
   1) Non-selective
   2) Indirect sympathomimetic activity (ISA); less cardiac depression at rest
   3) Adverse effects as above
e. Timolol:
   1) Nonselective
   2) A drug of choice in open angle glaucoma
   3) Adverse effects as above

3. ALPHA-ADRENERGIC RECEPTOR BLOCKING AGENTS: (See Chapter 2)

   a. Adverse effects, such as orthostatic hypotension, tachycardia, etc., have made general alpha-adrenergic blocking drugs clinically unacceptable for treating hypertension.
   b. Exception: May be useful during surgical removal of pheochromocytoma to prevent excessive hypertension caused by the release of catecholamines during surgical manipulation of the tumor.
   c. Prazosin: Newer antihypertensive drug which acts selectively on the post-synaptic alpha$_1$ receptor of vascular smooth muscle. Orthostatic hypotension and reflex tachycardia are not as prominent as with other alpha-blockers. May have some CNS sympatho-inhibiting action.

4. MIXED ANTAGONIST:

   Labetalol: (See details in Chapter 2).

5. ADRENERGIC NEURON BLOCKERS:

   a. Reserpine:
      1) Depletes NE stores by preventing uptake and storage in neurosecretory granules - appears to act by inhibiting transport and binding of catecholamines in storage granules; depletes both in peripheral sympathetics and in the brain.
      2) Get unopposed parasympathetic effects - bradycardia, nasal stuffiness, GI effects (diarrhea, increased motility, aggravation of peptic ulcers).
      3) Other adverse effects: excessive sedation, depression, extrapyramidal symptoms, impotence.
   b. Guanethidine:
      1) Complex actions on the adrenergic neuron; prevents NE release when nerve is stimulated by blocking transmission of the action potential into the terminal nerve ending; also can deplete peripheral stores of NE and block reuptake of NE; does not cross blood-brain-barrier; no CNS effect.
      2) Slow onset (2-3 days) with long duration of action (effects persist for about a week after drug is stopped).
      3) Causes postural hypotension, bradycardia, diarrhea, nasal stuffiness, failure of ejaculation.

6. GANGLIONIC BLOCKING AGENTS:

   a. Hypotensive action is primarily due to reduced vasomotor tone, decreased venous return and lowered cardiac output
   b. Now rarely used because of side effects
   c. Trimethaphan: Occasionally used for hypertensive crisis; given by slow i.v. drip; dangerous drug - can cause precipitous fall in blood pressure; also may cause histamine release.

C. DIRECT VASODILATORS

1. ARTERIAL VASODILATORS (potassium channel activation = hyperpolarization and vascular smooth muscle relaxation)
   a. Hydralazine:
     1) Direct relaxant of vascular smooth muscle to decrease peripheral resistance.
     2) Reflex cardiac stimulation (increased cardiac output and tachycardia) can be blocked by administration of propranolol.
     3) Well absorbed after oral administration and generally well tolerated for treatment of chronic hypertension; useful in acute hypertensive crisis (parenteral).
     4) Adverse effects: Headache, palpitations, GI disturbances; most serious toxicity is a lupus-like syndrome occurring with long term therapy; this is reversible if drug stopped: this side effect limits its chronic use.
   b. Minoxidil:
     1) Long acting direct dilator of vascular smooth muscle.
     2) Reflex cardiac stimulation.
     3) Adverse effects: salt and water retention and hypertrichosis (growth of hair).
     4) Reserved for more severe and uncontrollable hypertension.
   c. Diazoxide:
     1) A non-diuretic congener of the thiazide diuretic drugs.
     2) Precise mechanism of action unknown, but exerts direct effect on the arterioles to lower blood pressure.
     3) Given i.v. for acute hypertensive emergencies.
     4) Adverse effects: Hyperglycemia (inhibits insulin release from the beta cells of the pancreas), hyperuricemia, amylase elevations and even pancreatic necrosis.

2. CALCIUM CHANNEL ANTAGONISTS:

   a. Consider for monotherapy.
   b. Nifedipine: most potent vasodilator but also most potent reflex cardiac effects.
   c. Others act more directly on heart to limit reflex cardiac effects.
   d. Poor choice of drug in patients with aortic stenosis or severe heart failure.

3. ARTERIAL AND VENOUS VASODILATOR:

    a. <u>Sodium nitroprusside</u>:
       1) An older drug, long considered obsolete has recently been revived
       2) A direct peripheral vasodilator and causes marked hypotension when administered i.v.
       3) Used in acute hypertensive emergencies, not considered suitable for chronic management of hypertension.
       4) Hazardous - can precipitate marked hypotension; light sensitive. Metabolized to thiocyanate; may cause psychotic syndrome.

D. CONVERTING ENZYME INHIBITORS

1. CAPTOPRIL:
    a. Inhibits the formation of angiotensin II and prevents the degradation of bradykinin.
    b. Also lowers blood pressure in "low-renin" patients.
    c. Orally effective; approved for monotherapy; also used to treat CHF (congestive heart failure) and diagnosis of renovascular disease.

2. ENALAPRIL:
    a. Action like captopril but more potent and longer acting.
    b. Prodrug; hydrolyzed in body to enalaprilat, an active metabolite.
    c. Maximum plasma levels of oral enalapril reached in 3-4 hrs; i.v. enalaprilat acts in 15 min.

3. LISINOPRIL:

    a. Newer ACE inhibitor that is orally effective when administered once/day.
    b. Onset of action about one hour; minimal side effects include dizziness, headache, fatigue and diarrhea.

REVIEW QUESTIONS

ONE BEST ANSWER

1. The following drug fails to prevent angina resulting from coronary artery spasm:

   A. Nitroglycerin
   B. Nifedipine
   C. Verapamil
   D. Nicardipine
   E. Propranolol

2. The following drug may increase the ventricular heart rate when atrial fibrillation is present:

   A. Diltiazem
   B. Propranolol
   C. Flecainide
   D. Quinidine
   E. Digoxin

3. A decrease in the QT interval of the surface electrocardiogram can be observed following the administration of:

   A. Bretylium
   B. Disopyramide
   C. Encainide
   D. Mexiletine
   E. Amiodarone

4. Negative inotropy and chronotropy are most prominent with which one of the following calcium antagonists:

   A. Nifedipine
   B. Nicardipine
   C. Isradipine
   D. Diltiazem
   E. Verapamil

5. Nicardipine reduces myocardial oxygen consumption by:

   A. Decreasing the sinus heart rate
   B. Increasing the sinus heart rate
   C. Increasing left ventricular preload
   D. Decreasing left ventricular afterload
   E. Decreasing myocardial contractility

6. A hemodynamic action of propranolol which is detrimental to its ability to reduce myocardial oxygen consumption is:

   A. Sinus bradycardia
   B. Sinus tachycardia
   C. Increased left ventricular preload
   D. Decreased left ventricular preload
   E. Coronary artery dilatation

7. Which one of the following statements is true concerning the action of enalapril?

   A. Prodrug for an angiotensin II receptor blocker
   B. Stimulates angiotensin receptors
   C. Increases endogenous bradykinin levels
   D. Does not effectively lower blood pressure in "normal renin" hypertensive patients

8. Which one of the following mechanisms best explains the antihypertensive actions of clonidine?

   A. Blockade of B_1-adrenergic receptors
   B. Blockade of CNS α-adrenergic receptors
   C. Stimulation of CNS α-adrenergic receptors
   D. Blockade of peripheral α-adrenergic receptors
   E. Stimulation of peripheral α-adrenergic receptors

9. A syndrome resembling systemic lupus erythematosus occurs in about 10% of patients receiving moderate to high doses of which one of the following antihypertensive drugs?

   A. Hydralazine
   B. Hydrochlorothiazide
   C. Diazoxide
   D. Sodium nitroprusside
   E. Guanethidine

80

ONE BEST ANSWER

10. Which one of the following would most likely increase plasma renin activity?

   A. Blood transfusion
   B. α-Methyldopa
   C. Propranolol
   D. Chlorothiazide
   E. Metaprolol

11. Changes commonly observed after digitalization of a patient with congestive heart failure may include all of the following EXCEPT:

   A. An increase in myocardial contractile force
   B. A marked increase in cardiac output
   C. A decrease in central venous pressure
   D. A decrease in blood pressure
   E. A decrease in heart rate

12. The usefulness of a cardiac glycoside in the management of atrial fibrillation depends upon its ability to:

   A. Decrease the rate of atrial impulse formation
   B. Decrease vagal control over the heart
   C. Decrease conduction time through the A-V node
   D. Increase the effective refractory period of the A-V node
   E. Increase conduction time in the atria

13. In the normal individual, digitalis can cause all of the following EXCEPT:

   A. Constriction of arteriolar smooth muscle
   B. Constriction of venous smooth muscle
   C. Diuresis
   D. Reduction of the venous return to the heart
   E. Sinus tachycardia

14. Cardiac glycosides are most effective in the treatment of heart failure caused by:

   A. Arteriovenous fistula
   B. Essential hypertension
   C. Anemia
   D. Thyrotoxicosis
   E. Diphtheria

15. All of the following actions may be observed in a patient with congestive heart failure after digitalization EXCEPT:

   A. Premature ventricular contractions (extrasystoles)
   B. Shortening of the P-R interval of the EKG
   C. Depression of the S-T segment of the EKG
   D. Slowing of conduction through the A-V node
   E. Inversion of the T wave of the EKG

16. Cardiac glycoside toxicity is enhanced by which ONE of the following:

   A. Decreased extracellular Ca^{++}
   B. Decreased stimulation rate
   C. Increased extracellular Mg^{++}
   D. Decreased extracellular K^+
   E. Decreased extracellular Na^+

17. All of the following can be used rationally to augment cardiac glycoside therapy of congestive heart failure EXCEPT:

   A. Vasodilators to decrease afterload
   B. Treat the underlying cause of the heart failure
   C. Diuretics to help decrease edema and volume overload
   D. Raise serum K^+ to extend therapeutic range of the glycoside
   E. ACE inhibitors to reduce both the preload and afterload

18. All of the following are true of digoxin EXCEPT:

   A. Is well absorbed after oral administration (up to 75%)
   B. Has a rapid onset of action
   C. Has a half-life of about five to seven days
   D. Is primarily excreted unchanged by the kidney
   E. Has the same potential (therapeutic index) for toxicity as digitoxin

19. All of the following are true of cholestyramine EXCEPT:

   A. Lowers LDL and plasma cholesterol
   B. May interfere with the absorption of warfarin
   C. Compliance is a problem because of its unpleasant taste and smell
   D. Decreases the synthesis of cholesterol
   E. Benefits have been demonstrated in CAHD

ONE BEST ANSWER

20. Nicotinamide:

A. Lowers both cholesterol and triglycerides
B. Contraindicated in a high risk patient with CAHD
C. Reduces LDL synthesis
D. Inhibits triglyceride lipase activation by lipolytic hormones
E. Is just as effective as nicotinic acid as a vitamin

MATCHING: use each letter only once.

Match the following drugs with the most appropriate side effects.

A. Minoxidil
B. Reserpine
C. Hydralazine
D. Diazoxide
E. Clonidine

21. Lupus-like syndrome

22. Hyperglycemia

23. Hypertrichosis

24. Sedation and increased G.I. motility

25. Rebound hypertension on drug withdrawal

MATCHING: Use each letter only once.

A. Prazosin   D. Atenolol
B. Pindolol   E. Metaprolol
C. Nadolol   F. Labetalol

26. Once per day administration due to long half-life

27. Intrinsic sympathomimetic activity

28. "Cardioselective", mainly renal elimination

29, "Cardioselective", mainly hepatic elimination

30. α- and ß-Adrenoceptor blockade

31. α-1 Adrenoceptor selective

MATCHING: Use each letter only once

Match the following drugs with the most appropriate mechanism of action.

A. Amrinone   F. Lisinopril
B. Cholestyramine   G. Lovastatin
C. Digoxin   H. Minoxidil
D. Dobutamine   I. Nicotinic acid
E. Gemfibrozil   J. Nitroprusside

32. Positive inotropic agent that inhibits phosphodiesterase

33. Positive inotropic agent that inhibits Na^+/K^+-ATPase

34. Ion-exchange resin that binds bile acids in the gut

35. Inhibits the rate-limiting enzyme in cholesterol synthesis (HMG-CoA reductase)

36. Inhibits angiotensin converting enzyme

MATCHING: A letter may be used more than once or not at all.

From the list below, select the drug most closely associated with the toxicity/side effect below.

A. Amiodarone   E. Nitroglycerin
B. Nifedipine   F. Verapamil
C. Furosemide   G. Procainamide
D. Flecainide   H. Acetazolamide

37. Pedal edema

38. Torsades de pointes

39. Drug-induced lupus erythematosus

40. Hyperuricemia

41. Hyperthyroidism/hypothyroidism

42. Hypokalemia

43. May precipitate congestive heart failure

44. Corneal opacities

MATCHING: A letter can be used more than once or not at all.

From the list below select the drug which is most closely associated with the drug action/effect listed below.

A. Aldosterone
B. Triamterene
C. Bretylium
D. Spironolactone
E. Propranolol
F. Disopyramide
G. Flecainide
H. Hydrochlorothiazide

I. Nifedipine
J. Lisinopril
K. Lidocaine
L. Acetazolamide
M. Mannitol
N. Nitroglycerin
O. Diltiazem

45. Competitive inhibitor of aldosterone at the aldosterone receptor

46. Reduces the enzymatic formation of angiotensin II from angiotensin I

47. Prolongs ventricular muscle action potential duration without slowing conduction velocity

48. Increase action potential duration and slows conduction velocity in ventricular tissue

49. Slows conduction velocity in all cardiac tissues, regardless of heart rate

50. Slows conduction only in slow response cardiac tissues (AV node and sinus node)

51. Reduces myocardial oxygen consumption by reducing the sinus heart rate and myocardial contractility.

52. Slows conduction velocity in rapid response tissues only at rapid heart rates

53. Produces a dramatic decrease in myocardial preload by dilating venous capacitance vessels

54. Reduces slow inward current in ventricular myocardium

55. May facilitate conduction through the AV node by competitive blockade of muscarinic receptors

56. Blocks the increase in heart rate and contractility observed with nitroglycerin administration

57. Reduces glucose tolerance and may precipitate frank hyperglycemia in some patients

58. Reduces the mortality from sudden death following myocardial infarction

CHAPTER 5: DRUGS AFFECTING HEMOSTASIS AND HEMATOPOIESIS

I. DRUGS WHICH AFFECT BLOOD COAGULATION

Injury to blood vessels results in a series of events aimed at preventing blood loss (hemostasis), which include vasoconstriction, platelet aggregation, and the deposition of fibrin. THROMBOSIS can be defined as the inappropriate response of the hemostatic process to alterations in the circulatory system, lesions in vascular walls, or other stimuli. EMBOLISM occurs when thrombi are dislodged and are carried by the circulation to small vessels, where they may cause occlusions and tissue ischemia. Thrombosis is treated by pharmacological intervention designed to inhibit platelet function, inhibit fibrin deposition, or to enhance fibrinolysis.

A. DRUGS WHICH INHIBIT PLATELET FUNCTION (Antithrombic Drugs)

Aspirin	Dipyridamole
Sulfinpyrazone	Ticlopidine

When platelets are stimulated to aggregate, arachidonic acid is liberated from platelet phospholipids, and may be metabolized to thromboxane A_2 by the sequential actions of cyclooxygenase and thromboxane synthetase. As this occurs, platelet levels of cyclic AMP decrease, and ADP is released. Both ADP and thromboxane A_2 are potent stimuli for platelet aggregation.

1. ASPIRIN acetylates platelet cyclooxygenase and irreversibly inhibits the enzyme. Aspirin is usually given at a dose of 325 mg per day for its antithrombic effects. Major adverse effects include GI distress and bleeding.

2. SULFINPYRAZONE has a less reliable antithrombic effect than aspirin, but does not cause bleeding abnormalities. It may reversibly inhibit cyclooxygenase activity.

3. DIPYRIDAMOLE inhibits platelet ADP release by increasing cyclic AMP levels, through two apparent mechanisms. Dipyridamole increases adenosine concentrations in the blood, which stimulates adenyl cyclase. Dipyridamole is also a phosphodiesterase inhibitor, and slows cyclic AMP catabolism. Dipyridamole also decreases the adhesion of platelets to artificial surfaces.

4. TICLOPIDINE inhibits ADP-induced platelet fibrinogen binding and subsequent platelet-platelet interactions. Ticlopidine is indicated for patients who have experienced thrombotic stroke or stroke precursors, and is recommended for patients who cannot take aspirin.

B. DRUGS WHICH DECREASE FIBRIN FORMATION (Anticoagulants)

Heparin   Oral Anticoagulants   Enoxaparin

1. HEPARIN is an endogenous sulfated mucopolysaccharide found in mast cells bound to histamine. The drug is commercially prepared from pork stomach and beef lung. Heparin combines with, and catalytically activates, a plasma cofactor named antithrombin-III. This complex neutralizes several activated clotting factors, particularly factors IIa (thrombin) and Xa. Heparin is active to a lesser extent against activated forms of factors VIII, IX, XI, and XII. It has no therapeutic effects other than the inhibition of clotting. Heparin causes the release of lipoprotein lipase from tissues, which hydrolyzes plasma triglycerides and has a "clearing" effect on turbid plasma.

   a. Absorption, Fate and Excretion:
      1) Poor oral absorption; given i.v. or s.c. Do not give i.m.
      2) Duration of action; 2-4 hours
      3) Dosage is adjusted according to coagulation time (activated partial thromboplastin time) in therapy of acute thrombotic episodes. For prophylaxis, low doses of heparin are given which cause little change in clotting time.
      4) Dosage expressed in units (1 mg is approximately 100 units)
      5) Main metabolic fate is uptake by macrophages and endothelial cells. Some liver metabolism and urinary excretion also occur.
   b. Adverse Effects:
      1) Hemorrhage. PROTAMINE SULFATE is an antidote for heparin, and forms a 1:1 complex with the anticoagulant.
      2) Thrombocytopenia. May be mild and transient, or severe if anti-platelet antibodies are formed.
      3) Osteoporosis, when long-term heparin therapy is necessary.
      4) Allergy, probably develops to animal proteins in the solution.

2. ENOXAPARIN is a low molecular weight heparin which also binds antithrombin-III, but the complex is less effective than the heparin-activated complex against thrombin. As a result, enoxaparin exerts an antithrombotic effect (primarily attributed to inhibition of clotting factor Xa), but has little effect on bleeding time.

   a. Absorption, Fate and Excretion:
      1) Given by s.c. injection
      2) Enoxaparin is less susceptible to degradation by platelet factor 4 than heparin, and has a longer half-life. The usual dose is 30 mg every 12 hours.

b. Adverse effects:
  1) Contraindicated in patients with major bleeding.
  2) May produce mild thrombocytopenia, and periodic platelet counts should be taken.
  3) Cannot be used interchangeably (unit for unit) with heparin or other low molecular weight heparin preparations.

3. ORAL ANTICOAGULANTS include the coumarin (WARFARIN) and indanedione (anisindione) derivatives. Individual drugs within these chemical groups differ only in the onset and duration of action. The oral anticoagulant drugs antagonize the hepatic synthesis of the vitamin K-dependent clotting factors II (prothrombin), VII, IX and X. They have an onset of action of 2-3 days, during which time pre-existing levels of clotting factors are diminished. Other vitamin K-dependent functions may be affected as well; for example, this may explain the teratogenic effects of these drugs.

  a. Absorption, Fate and Excretion
    1) Well absorbed after oral administration
    2) Highly bound to plasma proteins (>90%)
    3) Metabolized in liver prior to excretion
    4) Highly variable effects from patient to patient. Adjust dosage on basis of prothrombin time.
  b. Adverse Effects:
    1) Hemorrhage
    2) Teratogenesis, especially during first trimester
    3) Liver and kidney toxicity - seen only with indanedione derivatives and limits the usefulness of this chemical class of anticoagulants
    4) Drug interactions occur between the oral anticoagulants and many other drugs.
  c. Oral anticoagulant antagonist : PHYTONADIONE (vitamin K_1)

C. THROMBOLYTIC DRUGS promote the dissolution of thrombi by stimulating the conversion of endogenous plasminogen to plasmin (fibrinolysin). Bleeding is the primary adverse effect of these drugs. Patients may also require anticoagulant therapy to prevent reocclusion of blood vessels.

  1. STREPTOKINASE is produced from cultures of beta-hemolytic streptococci and is therefore antigenic, but readily available. Allergic and febrile reactions are the most common non-hemorrhagic side effects.

  2. ANISTREPLASE is an acylated plasminogen-streptokinase activator complex. It is activated after deacylation in the body. This combination is similar to streptokinase, but has a longer duration of thrombolytic action.

  3. UROKINASE is obtained from human urine or kidney tissue culture and is not antigenic, but is quite expensive.

4. TISSUE PLASMINOGEN ACTIVATOR (TPA) is a human protein, derived through the use of recombinant DNA methods. TPA is said to preferentially activate plasminogen bound to fibrin, which could result in "clot-specific" thrombolytic activity.

D. MISCELLANEOUS DRUGS WHICH ARE USED TO AFFECT HEMOSTASIS

1. AMINOCAPROIC ACID and TRANEXAMIC ACID inhibit plasmin and plasminogen activator. They can be used as antidotes to bleeding which occurs with thrombolytic therapy, and as adjuncts in the treatment of hemophiliacs.

2. DESMOPRESSIN (antidiuretic hormone) stimulates the release of clotting factor VIII from the vascular endothelium and may be used preoperatively in hemophilic patients with low circulating levels of this factor.

3. DIHYDROERGOTAMINE MESYLATE is a vasoconstricting agent (see drugs used in the treatment of migraine headaches) which accelerates venous return and thereby antagonizes vascular stasis. It is used alone or with heparin for prevention of postoperative deep vein thrombosis and pulmonary embolism.

4. PENTOXIFYLLIN is a dimethylxanthine derivative which decreases blood viscosity and increases erythrocyte flexibility. It is indicated in for intermittent claudication associated with occlusive arterial diseases of the limbs.

5. APROTININ is a protease inhibitor from beef lung which has hemostatic properties because it inhibits plasmin and kallikrein. It is used to reduce blood loss and the need for transfusions in patients undergoing coronary artery bypass graft procedures.

II. ANTI-ANEMIA DRUGS (HEMATINICS)

A. IRON DEFICIENCY ANEMIA

Iron is absorbed only in limited quantities from the small intestine and most of the absorption occurs in the duodenum and proximal jejunum. The drug of choice for treatment of iron deficiency anemia is ferrous sulfate, given 3 to 4 times per day, preferably on an empty stomach to increase iron absorption. Orally administered iron is associated with a high incidence of gastrointestinal symptoms, resulting from a direct toxic effect of iron. Patient non-compliance because of the GI symptoms is the most common cause of therapeutic failure. This problem can usually be resolved by an adjustment in dosage.

Iron Dextran may be given by IM or IV (preferred) injection. Dosages must be carefully calculated so that the body's storage capacity is not exceeded ("iron overload"). Parenterally administered iron is associated with a number of adverse effects and is indicated only when the need for iron cannot be met by oral administration.

Deferoxamine mesylate is a specific chelating agent for iron. It may be administered orally or parenterally for treatment of acute iron poisoning or iron overload.

B. FOLIC ACID DEFICIENCY

Folic acid is widely available in the diet, and deficiency due to dietary insufficiency alone is uncommon in the U.S. Alcohol and some drugs (e.g. anti-convulsants) are folate antagonists and may exacerbate megaloblastic anemia caused by folate deficiency. Folic acid is necessary for the biosynthesis of thymidylate and subsequent formation of DNA. Orally administered folic acid is usually adequate for all folate-deficient conditions.

Leucovorin (folinic acid) is injected to "rescue" normal cells after high-dose methotrexate treatment in cancer chemotherapy. Leucovorin can also be given as a folate supplement if oral therapy is not feasible.

C. CYANOCOBALAMIN (VITAMIN B_{12}) DEFICIENCY

The daily requirement for vitamin B_{12} is extremely low (2-5 µg), and because this vitamin is found in many foods of animal origin, a deficiency due to dietary insufficiency is rare. However, the absorption of vitamin B_{12} from the gastrointestinal tract requires the presence of a protein secreted in the stomach, intrinsic factor. The absence of intrinsic factor, as in pernicious anemia, results in inadequate vitamin B_{12} absorption.

Vitamin B_{12} is required for the normal metabolism of folic acid, and a B_{12} deficiency will cause a megaloblastic anemia because of diminished folate-dependent DNA synthesis. However, neurological symptoms observed in pernicious anemia apparently develop from defective biosynthesis of myelin, which does not involve folic acid.

CYANOCOBALAMIN or HYDROXOCOBALAMIN are normally given intramuscularly in the treatment of pernicious anemia, and treatment must be continued at monthly intervals for the rest of the patient's life. Oral vitamin B_{12} preparations with intrinsic factor derived from animals give erratic and unreliable results.

ERYTHROPOIETIN (Epoetin alpha) is a renal hormone which regulates the production of red blood cells in the bone marrow. Patients with chronic renal failure develop anemia secondary to inadequate levels of erythropoietin. Human recombinant erythropoietin has been shown to be effective in treatment of anemia associated with uremia. There are no direct adverse effects of replacement therapy, although about 25% of patients experience hypertension during treatment (mechanism not understood).

D. OTHER BLOOD MODIFIERS

Filagrastim (G-CSF)   Sargramostim (GM-CSF)

Granulocyte (G) and granulocyte-macrophage (GM) colony stimulating factors (CSF) are naturally occurring peptide growth factors. Their uses include stimulation of bone marrow growth after transplantation or cancer chemotherapy.

REVIEW QUESTIONS

ONE BEST ANSWER

1. If a patient is suffering from a megaloblastic anemia, and studies of the blood and urine indicate abnormally high concentrations of methylated folic acid derivatives, this would indicate that the patient is deficient in:

   A. Dihydrofolate reductase
   B. Dietary folic acid
   C. Cobalamin (vitamin B_{12})
   D. Transferrin
   E. Pyridoxine

2. Recombinant human erythropoietin has replaced androgens for the treatment of:

   A. Aplastic anemia
   B. Anemia associated with renal failure
   C. Anemia of chronic disease
   D. Sickle cell anemia
   E. Thalassemias

3. Anemia and neurological complications are symptoms of a deficiency of:

   A. Iron
   B. Pyridoxine
   C. Folic acid
   D. Cobalamin (vitamin B_{12})
   E. Thiamine

4. The anticoagulant action of heparin can be effectively counteracted by:

   A. Vitamin C
   B. Vitamin K
   C. Thromboplastin
   D. EDTA
   E. Protamine

5. The anticoagulant action of bishydroxycoumarin can be effectively counteracted by:

   A. Vitamin C
   B. Vitamin K
   C. Thromboplastin
   D. EDTA
   E. Protamine

MATCHING: Use each letter only once.

From the list below select the drug which is most closely associated with the action/effect listed below.

A. Aminocaproic acid
B. Anisindione
C. Aspirin
D. Desmopressin
E. Dipyridamole
F. Enoxaparin
G. Heparin
H. Pentoxifyllin
I. Streptokinase
J. Sulfinpyrazone
K. Tissue plasminogen activator
L. Warfarin

6. Increases erythrocyte flexibility and decreases blood viscosity

7. Stimulates vascular endothelial cells to release clotting factor VIII

8. Rapid acting anticoagulant which antagonizes the action of several clotting factors

9. Antigenic enzyme used in thrombolytic therapy

10. Hemostatic agent which is useful if excessive bleeding accompanies urokinase administration

11. In theory, could promote "clot-specific" thrombolysis

12. Reversible inhibitor of platelet cyclooxygenase activity

13. Orally effective anticoagulant, but causes renal and hepatic toxicity

14. Low molecular weight heparin derivative.

CHAPTER 6: DRUGS ACTING ON THE CENTRAL NERVOUS SYSTEM

I. ANESTHETIC AGENTS

A. GENERAL ANESTHETICS

1. GENERAL CONCEPTS:

a. Ideal Anesthetic: produces unconsciousness, analgesia and muscle relaxation; most anesthetics are not ideal anesthetics and are administered in combination with other preoperative medications.
b. Many types of compounds with varied structures can produce anesthesia; thus, anesthetic agents are not believed to produce their effects by interacting with specific receptors.
c. The lipid solubility of compounds is an important determinant of anesthetic potency.
d. Anesthetic agents prevent neuronal transmission by disrupting neuronal membrane structure and function.
e. Synaptic transmission is more susceptible to general anesthetics than axonal transmission.
f. Finely diverging neural networks in the CNS particularly are sensitive to general anesthetics, including the:
   1) Substantia Gelatinosa of the Spinal Cord Dorsal Horn: Termination site of primary afferents conveying painful information from the periphery to the CNS.
   2) Sensory Nuclei of the Thalamus: Supraspinal sites where painful information is processed.
   3) Reticular Formation: Regions of the brainstem that maintain consciousness and alertness.

2. UPTAKE AND DISTRIBUTION OF INHALATION ANESTHETICS:

a. The depth of anesthesia depends on the concentration of anesthetic in the brain. The concentration gradient governs the rate of diffusion of anesthetic from the inspired air to the blood to the brain tissue.
b. Minimum Alveolar Concentration (MAC) = alveolar concentration at which 50% of the patients fail to respond to a standard surgical stimulus. The MAC value indicates the potency of an anesthetic.
c. Because of their lipid solubility, anesthetics distribute readily to fatty tissues, which then can act as reservoirs.

3. FACTORS INFLUENCING THE RATE OF INDUCTION OF INHALATION ANESTHETICS:

    a. <u>Concentration in inspired air</u>. Concentration of anesthetic usually is increased during induction; however, the irritability of the agent to the airways may be a limiting factor.

    b. <u>Ventilation rate and depth</u>. Increased ventilation rate and depth leads to an increased rate of induction.

    c. <u>Blood solubility</u>. Low solubility = rapid induction rate = rapid recovery rate. High solubility = slow induction rate = slow recovery rate.

    d. <u>Blood flow and cardiac output</u>. Uptake of anesthetic into tissues is dependent on blood flow.

4. SPECIFIC AGENTS:

    a. Volatile Liquids

       1) <u>Halothane</u>: Does not produce complete analgesia or muscle relaxation (often administered in combination with opioids or nitrous oxide and muscle relaxants); 80% of administered halothane is exhaled unchanged, 20% is metabolized by the liver and excreted; produces dose-dependent hypotension; sensitizes the myocardium to adrenergic agonists and may increase the likelihood of arrhythmias; can cause <u>malignant hyperthermia</u> in predisposed individuals, treat with <u>dantrolene</u>.

       2) <u>Isoflurane</u>: Commonly used anesthetic; similar to halothane; potentiates the effects of muscle relaxant; no hepatic or renal toxicity.

       3) <u>Enflurane</u>: Similar to halothane; minimal cardiovascular effects; may cause tonic/clonic muscular activity and seizures.

       4) <u>Methoxyflurane</u>: Most potent anesthetic available; fluoride toxicity prevents routine clinical use.

    b. Gaseous Agents
<u>Nitrous Oxide</u>: Good analgesic; does not produce deep anesthesia except with very high doses where oxygenation is inadequate; always administered with 30-35% oxygen; <u>second gas effect</u> -- massive outflow of gas into the alveoli upon termination of the anesthetic, oxygen must be administered; long-term exposure to trace concentrations may cause pernicious anemia and an increased incidence of spontaneous abortions.

    c. Intravenous Agents

       1) <u>Thiopental</u>: Ultra-short acting barbiturate; induction agent; hypnosis occurs in 30-60 sec; action of a bolus dose is terminated by redistribution to other tissues; metabolized by liver; may cause myocardial and respiratory depression.

       2) <u>Diazepam</u>: Benzodiazepine; induction agent; minimal cardiovascular effects, produces NO analgesia; high incidence of phlebitis.

       3) <u>Midazolam</u>: Benzodiazepine; similar to diazepam; greater water solubility; less irritating; short onset of action; more rapid elimination.

4) <u>Ketamine</u>: Dissociative anesthetic; produces cardiovascular stimulation and increased intracranial pressure; use is limited clinically because of hallucinations following recovery.

B. LOCAL ANESTHETICS

1. GENERAL CONCEPTS:

a. Local anesthetics <u>reversibly</u> block nerve conduction; they do <u>not</u> produce hypnosis or sedation.
b. Agents must have both lipophilic and hydrophilic properties to be effective by parenteral injection; most are weak bases.
c. Local anesthetics are classified as either <u>esters</u> or <u>amides</u>.
d. In the body local anesthetics exist in two forms: the uncharged base and the charged acid. Only the uncharged base can cross nerve membranes; however, once inside the nerve axon, it is the charged form that is active.
e. Tissue acidity (as occurs with inflammation and infection) can impede the development of local anesthesia.
f. Local anesthetics interfere with the <u>propagation</u> of action potentials in nerve axons by blocking sodium channels; blockade is usage and frequency dependent.

2. PHARMACOLOGIC AND ADVERSE EFFECTS:

a. Central Nervous System
1) Local anesthetics readily pass from the peripheral circulation into the brain because of their lipid solubility.
2) Local anesthetics can cause stimulation of the CNS if a sufficient amount of drug is absorbed from the injection site. Initial signs and symptoms of CNS toxicity include: dizziness, analgesia, numbness, visual and auditory disturbances. If blood levels are sufficiently high, convulsions can occur; treat with intravenous diazepam.
3) CNS stimulation is followed by respiratory and cardiovascular depression and a loss of consciousness.
b. Cardiovascular System
1) In toxic doses, local anesthetics can produce cardiovascular depression and circulatory collapse.
2) Some influences on the cardiovascular system can be beneficial (e.g., treatment of arrythmias). In non-toxic doses, local anesthetics increase the effective refractory period and decrease cardiac automaticity.
3) Local anesthetics inhibit myogenic activity and autonomic tone and produce vasodilation in the area of injection.
c. Hypersensitivity
1) Occurs most commonly with <u>ester</u> local anesthetics
2) Reaction may manifest itself as an allergic dermatitis or an asthmatic attack.

3. VASOCONSTRICTORS:

   a. Vasoconstrictors are added to local anesthetic solutions to decrease systemic absorption and prolong the duration of action.
   b. Clinically, epinephrine is considered to be the most effective.
   c. Vasoconstrictors should be used with caution in patients with cardiac disease, high blood pressure, hyperthyroidism and other vascular diseases.

4. ABSORPTION, DISTRIBUTION AND EXCRETION:

   a. The rate of absorption is dependent on the: dosage, presence of a vasoconstrictor, nature of the administration site, and pharmacologic profile of the drug.
   b. Local anesthetics readily distribute to other tissues; redistribution is a major means for removal of amide local anesthetics from the blood.
   c. Ester local anesthetics primarily are inactivated by hydrolysis and eliminated in the urine.
   d. Amide local anesthetics primarily are metabolized by the liver involving N-dealkylation and hydrolysis; hepatic blood flow is the rate limiting factor; use with caution in patients with severe hepatic disease.

5. SPECIFIC AGENTS:

   a. Procaine: Prototype ester; short duration of action
   b. Lidocaine: Prototype amide; widely used, intermediate duration of action
   c. Cocaine: Produces vasoconstriction; high abuse potential; limited use for topical application to mucosa of nose and pharynx
   d. Benzocaine: Topical use only; poorly soluble in water
   e. Bupivacaine: Amide anesthetic; suitable for injection; long duration of action

6. TECHNIQUES OF ANESTHESIA ADMINISTRATION:

   a. Surface/Topical Application: Applied to skin or mucous membranes.
   b. Infiltration: Inject dilute solution and let diffuse (e.g., subcutaneous or submucosal).
   c. Nerve Block: Inject close to nerve trunk, but proximal to intended area of anesthesia (i.e., anesthetize nerve innervating area).
   d. Spinal: Inject anesthetic in subarachnoid space.
   e. Epidural: Inject within vertebral canal, but outside dura.

II. PAIN RELIEF

A. OPIOID AGONISTS

1. FUNCTIONAL CLASSIFICATION:

   a. <u>Agonists</u>: morphine, methadone, fentanyl, meperidine, oxycodone, codeine, propoxyphene, hydrocodone, heroin
   b. <u>Antagonists</u>: naloxone, naltrexone
   c. <u>Mixed Agonists/Antagonists</u>: pentazocine, butorphanol, nalbuphine, buprenorphine
   d. <u>Antitussives</u>: codeine, dextromethorphan
   e. <u>Antidiarrheals</u>: diphenoxylate, loperamide

2. CHEMISTRY:

   a. Small molecular alterations can alter the action of opioid compounds (i.e., agonists converted to antagonists); pharmacokinetic properties also can be altered significantly.
   b. Antagonist properties are associated with large groups on the nitrogen atom, such as allyl groups in the case of naloxone.

3. MECHANISM AND SITES OF ACTION:

   a. Five opioid receptors have been identified:
      1) <u>Mu</u>: mediate analgesia, sedation, miosis, euphoria, constipation, respiratory depression, physical dependence
      2) <u>Kappa</u>: mediate analgesia, miosis, sedation, dysphoria
      3) <u>Delta</u>: mediate affective behavior
      4) <u>Sigma</u>: mediate dysphoria, hallucinations
      5) <u>Epsilon</u>: mediate affective behavior
   b. Opioids have both spinal and supraspinal sites of action.
      1) Inhibit release of neurotransmitters from primary afferents.
      2) Activate descending inhibitory pathways which modulate pain transmission in the spinal cord.
      3) Modulate pain transmission in the thalamus and limbic system.

4. ENDOGENOUS OPIOIDS:

   a. Three families of endogenous opioid peptides have been identified:
      1) <u>Endorphins</u>: Parent protein is pro-opiomelanocortin; function as neurohormones; may mediate the psychological responses to pain and stress.
      2) <u>Enkephalins</u>: Precursor is proenkephalin A; found throughout the brain and spinal cord; function as neurotransmitters.
      3) <u>Dynorphins</u>: Precursor is prodynorphin; function as neurotransmitters.

b. Endogenous opioids do <u>not</u> play a significant role in normal pain reactions; they may become physiologically active in certain situations, and may explain acupuncture and the placebo phenomenon.

5. ORGAN SYSTEM EFFECTS OF OPIOIDS:

  a. Central Nervous System
1) <u>Analgesia</u>: Selective effect, other sensory modalities are unaffected; suppress both the perception and reaction to pain.
2) <u>Euphoria</u>: Commonly occurs when an indication for opioids exists; non-pain experiencing users may report dysphoria.
3) <u>Sedation</u>: Drowsiness and mental cloudiness can occur.
4) <u>Respiratory Depression</u>: Depression of brainstem respiratory mechanisms; decreased responsiveness of chemoreceptors to CO_2.
5) <u>Cough Suppression</u>: Suppression of the medullary cough reflex center.
6) <u>Emetic Action</u>: Initial doses can stimulate the chemoreceptor trigger zone in the medulla causing nausea and vomiting.
7) <u>Miosis (pinpoint pupils)</u>: Stimulation of the oculomotor nucleus; little or no tolerance develops to this effect.
8) <u>Truncal Rigidity</u>: Increased tone of large trunk muscles.

  b. Peripheral Effects
1) <u>Cardiovascular System</u>: Minimal effects at analgesic doses; IV administration can cause local histamine release and itching.
2) <u>Gastrointestinal Tract</u>: Increased resting tone and decreased propulsive activity can cause constipation.
3) <u>Sphincters</u>: Increased tone can lead to biliary colic and postoperative urinary retention.
4) <u>Uterus</u>: May prolong labor by reducing uterine tone.

6. CLINICAL USES OF OPIOIDS:

  a. <u>Analgesia</u>: Severe, dull, constant pain is better relieved than sharp, stabbing pain; provide symptomatic treatment only; pain relief increases with age due to decreased metabolism and clearance.
  b. <u>Anti-Tussive</u>: Cough suppression can be obtained at lower doses than those needed for analgesia.
  c. <u>Anti-Diarrheal</u>: Should not be used as substitutes for antibiotic therapy.
  d. <u>Adjunct Medications for Anesthesia</u>: Used as preoperative drugs because of their sedative, anxiolytic and analgesic properties; high potency opioids (e.g., fentanyl) can be used as primary anesthetics when it is desirable to minimize cardiovascular effects.

7. TOLERANCE:

  a. Tolerance develops to most effects, <u>except</u> to the miosis and constipation produced by opioids.

B. OPIOID ANTAGONISTS

1. Antagonists can reverse most of the effects produced by opioids, but do not reverse the anti-tussive effects produced by opioids.

2. Naloxone is the drug of choice to reverse respiratory depression caused by opioids and can be used as a diagnostic test for illicit opioid use.
   a. High affinity for mu receptors; acts by competitive inhibition.
   b. Half-life is shorter than morphine; multiple doses may be required to reverse the depressant effects of opioids.
   c. Effective only by IV route due to extensive first pass metabolism.

C. MIXED AGONISTS/ANTAGONISTS

1. Used to treat mild to moderate pain.

2. Act as partial agonists or competitive antagonists at the mu receptor; also may act at delta and kappa receptors.

3. Have abuse potentials comparable to opioid agonists.

4. Pentazocine, nalbuphine, butorphanol and buprenorphine are examples of mixed agonists/antagonists.

D. ANTI-MIGRAINE DRUGS

1. AGENTS USEFUL FOR ACUTE MIGRAINE ATTACKS

   a. SUMATRIPAN:
      1) A selective 5-HT_{1D} receptor agonist that blocks neurogenic inflammation in the trigeminal vascular system.
      2) Effective at any time during the attack.
      3) Also helps to relieve nausea and vomiting which accompany the attack.
      4) Usually given by i.m. injection; orally active forms are under development.
   b. ERGOTAMINE:
      1) An ergot alkaloid that causes intense vasoconstriction. Has partial agonist or antagonist activity against tryptaminergic, dopaminergic, and α-adrenergic receptors.
      2) Not used as an oxytocic because it tends to cause uterine spasm.
      3) Poorly absorbed after oral administration; can also be given by sublingual, rectal, and i.m. routes.
      4) Caffeine enhances both the absorption and the peripheral action of ergotamine.

      5) Limitations have been placed on the total dose of ergotamine that can be taken per attack and per week in order to prevent ergot poisoning.

      6) Contraindicated in pregnancy (class X).

   c. DIHYDROERGOTAMINE MESYLATE:

      1) Less effective than ergotamine for relief of acute migraine, but causes lower incidence of vomiting when injected.

  2. AGENTS USEFUL FOR PROPHYLAXIS OF MIGRAINE

   a. METHYSERGIDE:

      1) An ergot alkaloid derivative, not useful for acute migraine.

      2) Patients should be monitored for fibrotic complications, such as retroperitoneal or pleuropulmonary fibrosis.

   b. Propranolol is currently the drug of choice for migraine prophylaxis, but its mechanism of anti-migraine action is unknown.

   c. Amitriptyline, calcium blockers, and clonidine have been useful, but their mechanisms of action are also unknown.

  3. CLUSTER HEADACHES

   a. Like migraine headaches, cluster headaches have unknown etiology, but also appear to result from changes in brain blood flow.

   b. Prophylaxis is preferred; methysergide is the drug of choice.

   c. Drugs which are effective in terminating migraine are usually effective in terminating cluster headaches.

   d. Approximately 50 - 70% of cluster headaches can be terminated by inhalation of 100% oxygen.

III. SEDATIVE - HYPNOTICS

Certain general depressants of the CNS are used to relieve anxiety, to sedate or to induce sleep (hypnosis). The magnitude of their effects is dose-dependent. Besides their sedative, hypnotic and anxiolytic properties, as a class they also are characterized as to their properties as anticonvulsants, CNS muscle relaxants and anesthetics, as well as by their ability to develop physical dependence.

A. BENZODIAZEPINES

  1. Marketing strategies by the pharmaceutical industry, rather than differences in their pharmacology, primarily determine how the benzodiazepines are classified. Classification of some of these agents is as follows (underlined agents are important to remember):

Hypnotics: <u>Flurazepam</u>, estazolam <u>temazepam</u>, <u>triazolam</u>, and quazepam.
Anxiolytics: <u>Diazepam</u>, chlordiazepoxide, oxazepam, lorazepam, alprazolam and chlorazepate.
Anticonvulsant: Clonazepam
Anesthetic Agent: Midazolam.

2. <u>Mechanism of action</u>: The benzodiazepines increase the ionic conductance of the $GABA_A$ receptor by increasing the frequency of channel opening.

3. <u>Flumazenil</u> is a relatively specific competitive benzodiazepine antagonist. It has no activity <u>per se</u> but can antagonize the sedative actions of the benzodiazepines.

4. There is no evidence that one benzodiazepine is clinically superior to another. Higher doses are required for the therapy of panic or for phobia than the dose for anxiety. Many of these agents have common intermediates (nordiazepam or a halogenated nordiazepam) with long half-lives (50-120 hours). Substitution with a triazolo ring prevents the formation of a desmethyldiazepam analogue, and thus triazolo drugs have shorter half lives.

5. Tolerance develops but is variable. Tolerance to the antianxiety effects of the drug is less likely to develop than to the sedative-hypnotic effects. Thus, their effectiveness as sedative-hypnotics may last only about four months with continuous use while their antianxiety effectiveness could last a life time.

6. Physical dependence can occur; withdrawal symptoms are similar to those seen with withdrawal from the barbiturates.

7. Microsomal enzyme induction does not occur with benzodiazepines but they can induce ALA synthetase. Clinically important is their degree of protein binding which is in the range of 90-99% for all except alprazolam (70-80%) .

B. BARBITURATES

1. <u>Mechanism of action</u>: Barbiturates increase ionic conductance of the $GABA_A$ receptor by increasing the duration of channel opening. Lipid solubility affects the onset and duration of their action. The two most important substitutions on the barbiturate ring are sulfur (thio) at the C_2 position to increase their lipid solubility, for use as i.v. anesthetics (<u>thiopental</u>), and phenyl at the C_5 position (<u>phenobarbital</u>), for use as an anticonvulsant. These are no longer used as sedative-hypnotics.

2. Barbiturates induce cytochrome P-450 microsomal enzyme activity which increases the rate of their own metabolism and also of other drugs metabolized by this system. They also induce aminolevulinic acid (ALA) synthetase, the rate limiting step in heme biosynthesis. Thus, barbiturates are contraindicated in patients with acute intermittent porphyria, porphyria variegata or a positive family history of these porphyrias.

3. Tolerance develops to their sedative and hypnotic effects and true physical dependence occurs. However no tolerance develops to the lethal dose or to the anticonvulsant actions of barbiturates.

C. OTHER AGENTS

1. Buspirone: A 5-HT$_{1A}$ receptor agonist resulting in inhibition of dorsal raphe discharge. It exerts a selective anxiolytic action that has a slow therapeutic onset (action may be delayed up to two weeks). Buspirone is not effective in the therapy of panic disorder.
2. Hydroxyzine: An antihistamine with sedative-anxiolytic, antiemetic and slight atropine-like actions. It can be given i.m. and will lowers the seizure threshold. It is not used in patients with neurological diseases.
3. Chloral hydrate: Metabolized to trichloroethanol. Like barbiturates, it can induce the drug metabolizing enzyme system. It is contraindicated in patients with acute intermittent porphyria.
4. Propranolol: Propranolol has a unique action in that it is more effective for the therapy of performance anxiety than the benzodiazepines. It is not effective for therapy of any of the chronic anxieties.
5. Meprobamate, although not as safe as the benzodiazepines, is being used with increasing frequency in the elderly. This is occurring because federal drug laws regulating the prescription of benzodiazepines tend to discourage their use.
6. Most over-the-counter sleep aids contain antihistamines and/or scopolamine.
7. Ethanol is the most widely used sedative-hypnotic.

IV. ALCOHOLS

Alcohols belong to the sedative-hypnotic CNS depressant class of drugs. The mechanism of the actions of ethanol are not understood, but interactions with GABA receptors, N-methyl-D-aspartate receptors, and condensation with certain biogenic amines to form opioid-like products have all been proposed.

A. ACUTE ETHANOL INTOXICATION

1. PHARMACOLOGICAL EFFECTS:
   a. CNS Effects: Intoxication is correlated in time with blood concentrations of ethanol. Subclinical (to 0.01%); vision and judgement impairments (0.04%). Emotional instability (0.2%) with decreased inhibitions, muscular incoordination; confusion (0.3%) staggering gait, slurred speech; stupor (0.4%); coma and death (0.6%).
   b. Gastrointestinal: Increased saliva and gastric secretions. Direct irritation to gastric and buccal mucosa, emesis due to central effect on chemoreceptor trigger zone and irritation of gastric mucosa. Decreased absorption of folates.

c. <u>Endocrine actions</u>: Suppression of vasopressin secretion, increased ACTH, cortisol, and catecholamine secretion.
d. <u>Cardiovascular system</u>: Initial transient tachycardia and hypertension, probably due to epinephrine release. Later bradycardia, negative inotropic action and hypotension.
e. <u>Kidney</u>: Diuresis due to decreased vasopressin release, as well as consumption of fluids.
f. <u>Body temperature</u>: Poikilothermia-hypothermia.

2. ETHANOL ABSORPTION AND ELIMINATION:

Approximately 30% of ethanol is absorbed from the stomach, and the remainder is rapidly absorbed from the small intestine. Ethanol is distributed according to tissue water content. Approximately 1-3% of ethanol is eliminated in the lungs (pulmonary blood/alveolar air ratio = 2100/1, the basis of breath tests), 2-6% is excreted by the kidney, and the remainder is oxidized in the liver at a constant rate. The total elimination rate is approximately 8-10 gms/hr, or 15-18 mg/100 ml blood/hr. Hepatic alcohol dehydrogenase is the primary enzyme involved in ethanol metabolism. In the metabolism of ethanol to acetaldehyde, the availability of NAD limits the rate of reaction of alcohol dehydrogenase (ADH). Acetaldehyde is metabolized to aldehyde dehydrogenase (ALDH).

3. TREATMENT OF OVERDOSE:

Treatment is primarily supportive. Patients should be kept warm and respiratory assistance may be needed.

4. THERAPEUTIC USE OF ETHANOL:

Ethanol is used as a solvent, germicide and for several topical applications. The popular notion that alcohol is a remedy for various complaints has no therapeutic validity.

B. PATHOLOGY OF CHRONIC ETHANOL ABUSE

1. <u>CNS Effects</u>: Wernicke's Syndrome, Korsakoff's psychosis, cerebral and cerebellar atrophy, alcoholic polyneuropathy (treated with thiamine)
2. <u>Gastrointestinal</u>: Peptic ulcers, esophagitis, gastritis and pancreatitis.
3. <u>Liver</u>: Steatosis, hepatitis, cirrhosis
4. <u>Muscle</u>: Cardiomyopathy, skeletal muscle myopathy
5. <u>Fetus</u>: Fetal alcohol syndrome (more common with binge drinking)

C. TOXICOLOGY OF OTHER ALCOHOLS

1. <u>Methanol</u>: Metabolized by ADH at about one-fifth the rate of ethanol to formaldehyde and then to formic acid. Toxicity due to metabolic acidosis and blindness caused by optic nerve damage. Treatment: Suppress methanol metabolism by administering ethanol; bicarbonate to correct acidosis.
2. <u>Ethylene Glycol</u>: Metabolized to oxalic acid, causing systemic acidosis. Treatment same as for methanol.

D. DISULFIRAM (ANTABUSE)

Disulfiram is an inhibitor of AlDH which can produce high blood levels of acetaldehyde after ethanol ingestion. Acetaldehyde syndrome includes skin flush (vasodilation), pulsating headache, dyspnea, nausea, and sweating. Clinically, disulfiram may be useful to reinforce the desire to stop drinking alcohol.

V. NEUROLOGIC DRUGS

A. ANTIEPILEPTIC DRUGS

SEIZURE DISORDER	DRUG OF CHOICE	ALTERNATIVES
Partial including secondarily generalized	Carbamazepine or Phenytoin	Primidone or Phenobarbital
Generalized		
Typical absence	Ethosuximide	Valproate
Atypical absence	Valproate	Combination of valproate and ethosuximide
Myoclonic	Valproate	Clonazepam or Phenobarbital
Infantile spasms	Corticotropin (ACTH)	Corticosteroids
Clonic or tonic	Valproate	Phenytoin
Tonic-clonic	Carbamazepine or Phenytoin or Valproate	Phenobarbital
Atonic/Akinetic	Valproate	Clonazepam or Phenytoin
Recurrent febrile	Phenobarbital	
Status epilepticus	Diazepam Lorazepam	Phenytoin or Phenobarbital

The term epilepsy is a collective designation for a group of chronic CNS disorders characterized by recurrent abnormal discharges of CNS neurons. The abnormal discharge may be limited to a focus or encompass wide areas. Although the abnormal discharge may have no clinical manifestations, such discharge often leads to a <u>seizure</u>. The epileptic seizure takes many forms, ranging from brief cessations of responsiveness without loss of consciousness to <u>convulsions</u> with accompanying loss of consciousness.

The drugs of choice and alternates or follow-up drugs are listed for each seizure disorder. The problem with misdiagnosis or improper drug selection is that the epilepsy is generally made worse when non-efficacious antiepileptic drugs are used.

1. <u>CARBAMAZEPINE</u>: Indications include partial seizures, generalized tonic-clonic seizures and mixed seizure patterns which are unmanageable with other antiepileptic drugs. The control of partial seizures usually requires higher plasma concentrations than necessary for generalized seizures. Carbamazepine is the drug of choice for trigeminal neuralgias and is used to treat rapidly cycling manic-depressive episodes. Auto-induction of drug metabolizing enzymes occurs and it has an active epoxide metabolite; high risk patients are those with hematological problems. Adverse effects include cognitive impairment, difficulty in sleeping, emotional liability, and diplopia.

2. <u>VALPROATE</u>: This agent is the closest to a universal antiepileptic drug. Ethosuximide is still preferred as the initial drug for treatment of typical absence seizures because of the potential for hepatotoxicity with valproate. It increases brain levels of GABA at inhibitory synapses. Gastric upset and sedation are common side effects. As hepatic and blood toxicity can occur; the patient must be monitored. There may be an increased risk of spina bifida in the fetus of pregnant females taking this drug during the first trimester.

3. <u>PHENYTOIN</u>: Previously phenytoin was the most frequently used antiepileptic drug, but it has several adverse effects, including cognitive impairment in (a) attention, (b) problem solving, and (c) visual motor tasks. Many physicians have limited their use of phenytoin in children and young women because of the following **non-dose-related** adverse effects: hypertrichosis (which is a darkening and increase of body hair), coarsening of facial features (involving thickening of the bridge of the nose, thickening of the lips and heavier brow ridges) and gingival hyperplasia (which can be controlled with good oral hygiene).

   Therapeutic drug monitoring is necessary with phenytoin (follows full Michaelis-Menton kinetics). During pregnancy, plasma levels are monitored more closely because about 25% of the women need marked increases and another 25% need marked decreases in dosage to maintain a therapeutic concentration. **Dose-related** adverse effects include nystagmus, ataxia, lethargy and coma.

4. PHENOBARBITAL: The only seizure types where phenobarbital remains the drug of choice are neonatal and febrile seizures. Prophylactic use is being challenged because recent studies showed no decrease in reoccurrence rate of seizures but did show a decrease in measured intelligence. Initial sedation, mental dullness and ataxia are the most troublesome dose-related adverse effects. Non-dose-related adverse effects include impaired short-term memory and hyperactivity in children. Allergic dermatitis and exfoliative dermatitis (Stevens-Johnson syndrome) are rare idiosyncratic adverse effects.

5. PRIMIDONE: Has two active metabolites, phenobarbital and phenylethylmalonamide. Adverse effects are the same as for phenobarbital; phantom localized gingival pain also occurs.

6. ETHOSUXIMIDE: The drug of choice for absence seizures, especially in pregnancy. Most common dose-related adverse effects include gastric distress, anorexia, drowsiness, and headache. Idiosyncratic adverse effects are rare but have included paranoid psychosis and bone marrow depression.

7. CORTICOTROPIN: Indicated for infantile spasms. Adverse effects include hypertension, electrolyte imbalances, and osteoporosis.

8. CLONAZEPAM: A benzodiazepine; has efficacy for myoclonic, atonic, akinetic and absence seizures. Tolerance develops with wide individual variability. Drug holidays often required.

B. ANTIPARKINSONISM DRUGS

   Parkinsonism is a chronic, progressive degenerative disease of the CNS resulting from loss of neurons in the substantia nigra. The aim of therapy is to restore dopaminergic activity which alleviates many of the clinical features of the disorder. An alternative but complementary approach is to restore balance of cholinergic and dopaminergic influences in the basal ganglia with anticholinergic drugs.

1. DOPAMINERGIC DRUGS
   a. L-DOPA: A prodrug. Crosses the blood brain barrier with the leucine amino acid transport system and is decarboxylated to dopamine. Regulation of the dose is difficult. Peripheral adverse effect include nausea, hypotension, and a potential for cardiac arrhythmias. Its combination with a peripheral decarboxylase inhibitor, carbidopa, reduces the dosage variability of L-dopa and its absolute amount by about 75%; the incidence of nausea and vomiting also is reduced from 80% to 20%. The drug combination increases the incidence of adverse CNS toxicity (involuntary movements and mental changes progressing to psychotic episodes).

b. <u>AMANTADINE</u>: A <u>dopamine</u> <u>releaser or facilitator</u>. It is only effective when sufficient dopamine stores exist. Therefore, it is used in early stages of the disease or as an adjunct to L-DOPA to improve the central regulation of dopamine. Also amantadine is an antiviral agent used for influenza A viruses.

c. <u>BROMOCRIPTINE</u>: A <u>dopamine D$_2$ receptor agonist</u>. It is not as effective as L-DOPA and most commonly is used in mid to late stages of the disease when the L-DOPA-carbidopa combination is not controlling symptoms. Mental depression is a more common side effect than with other dopaminergic drugs.

    It is the drug of choice for lowering elevated prolactin levels and for the suppression of post-partum lactation, galactorrhea, and amenorrhea, oligomenorrhea and infertility which are induced by hyperprolactinemia. It is used as an adjunct in some cases of acromegaly.

d. <u>SELEGILINE</u>: This drug is a reversible inhibitor of monoamine oxidase B and there is evidence that it may slow the progression of the disease. Selegiline is not an effective drug to relieve established parkinson symptoms.

2. ANTICHOLINERGIC DRUGS

Anticholinergic drugs are used both as the initial drug for therapy and combined with L-DOPA to reduce the tremor and rigidity of Parkinsonism. They have little effect on bradykinesia. Several anticholinergic drugs can be used but the most common are <u>trihexyphenidyl</u> and <u>benztropine</u>. <u>Procyclidine</u> is used if rigidity is the presenting symptom. Adverse effects of anticholinergics (incidence of 30 to 50%), include dizziness, nervousness, dry mouth, mild nausea and blurred vision.

C. CNS MUSCLE RELAXANTS

1. CENTRALLY ACTIVE MUSCLE RELAXANTS

a. <u>BACLOFEN</u>: Is the drug of choice for spinal spasticity. It is ineffective for stroke or spasticity of cerebral origin. Baclofen, which is chlorophenyl gamma-aminobutyric acid (GABA) is an agonist at bicuculline-insensitive GABA receptors (GABA$_B$). Abrupt termination of baclofen therapy may cause anxiety and hallucinations, thus the drug should be gradually discontinued. Baclofen also is indicated for trigeminal neuralgia and atypical facial pain.

<u>Interferon beta-1β</u> is becoming the drug of choice for moderate relapsing-remitting forms of multiple sclerosis

b. <u>CYCLOBENZAPRINE</u>: This agent is a structural analogue of the tricyclic antidepressant, amitriptyline, but it has no mood elevating effect. Tolerance develops with continued use. It is indicated only for acute muscle spasm (trauma, inflammation, trismus). Adverse effects are like those for the other tricyclic antidepressants. Cyclobenzaprine should not be used in patients with hyperthyroidism or cardiovascular disease.

c. <u>DIAZEPAM</u>: This is the sedative-hypnotic most frequently used for muscle relaxation. Methocarbamol and carisoprodol are marketed by the pharmaceutical industry exclusively for muscle relaxation. Diazepam is used in both acute and chronic conditions of muscle spasm. In chronic conditions, diazepam is given until tolerance develops, making it no longer effective (often takes months for effect to be lost). At that point, the diazepam is withdrawn for a short period and then therapy is reinitiated. Diazepam acts at the GABA$_A$ receptor including those in the spinal cord. It is the drug of choice for the "stiff man" syndrome.

2. LOCALLY ACTIVE MUSCLE RELAXANTS

<u>Dantrolene</u>: Dantrolene interferes with the intramuscular release of calcium from the sarcoplasmic reticulum and calcium efflux but it has no effect on neural pathways. It has   efficacy for spasticity induced by spinal cord and cerebral injuries. Common side effects include muscle weakness, drowsiness, and nausea. It is not given to patients with amyotrophic lateral sclerosis.

Fatal hepatotoxicity has occurred with long term dantrolene therapy and with high doses. Patients receiving long-term dantrolene therapy should be monitored for hepatic damage (e.g., SGOT, SGPT).   Dantrolene is the drug of choice for prophylaxis and treatment of malignant hyperthermia, a familial multifactorial genetic deficiency in the ability of the sarcoplasmic reticulum to store calcium.

<u>Chymopapain</u>: Chymopapain is a proteolytic enzyme used in patients with sciatica caused by a herniated lumbar disc (injected directly into the disc),

VI. PSYCHOPHARMACOLOGIC DRUGS

A. CENTRAL NERVOUS SYSTEM STIMULANTS

1. <u>Amphetamines</u> are used to treat narcolepsy and attention deficit disorder (ADD). Tolerance does not develop to the beneficial effect of amphetamines in these disorders. <u>Methylphenidate</u> is preferred to <u>dextroamphetamine</u> in children because it has equal efficacy in the therapy of ADD without long term inhibition of growth. Several appetite suppressants, including amphetamines, have been used in the treatment of obesity. Tolerance to the appetite suppressant action of amphetamines develops rapidly, within a few week, and appetite control is lost despite continued use. Because separation of the central stimulant actions and the development of tolerance from the appetite suppressant effect of the drugs can not be achieved, the use of these agents for the treatment of obesity is limited and controversial.   Amphetamines are powerful CNS stimulants and are thought to be acting by the release of monoamines from storage sites in central neurons.

2. The methylxanthines, caffeine and theophylline, are effective for the treatment of apnea in the premature infant. The antisoporific action (increased wakefulness) of methylxanthines results from adenosine receptor antagonism. This is in contrast to the ability to of the methylxanthines to increase cyclic AMP levels and modulate intracellular calcium transport when used for asthma. They also are thought to act by releasing monoamines from central neurons. Tolerance develops to the central and other effects of these drugs.

3. Cocaine is a drug that has amphetamine-like central stimulant actions. Cocaine blocks the neuronal reuptake of monoamines and potentiates the actions of these biogenic amines both centrally and peripherally. Although cocaine is an excellent topical local anesthetic, its clinical use is very limited because of the widespread abuse of this agent.

B. ANTIDEPRESSANTS AND LITHIUM

The constellation of fatigue, musculoskeletal complaints, sleep disorder, and loss of joy in living is characteristic of depression. Tricyclic antidepressants and related drugs are used to treat endogenous depression (about 25% of all depressions). Reactive depression (greater than 60% prevalence) responds to a variety of ministrations. Bipolar affective depression (manic-depressive), about 10% prevalence, is treated with lithium or carbamazepine. Significant clinical improvement, and not complete recovery, is considered successful treatment for endogenous depression. At least one third of patients treated with tricyclic antidepressants will fail to respond. A minimum three week trial is required before a change in dosage should be considered.

1. TRICYCLIC ANTIDEPRESSANTS

Tricyclic antidepressants are structurally related to phenothiazines but the three dimensional orientation of the phenyl rings is altered because of changes in the center ring. Thus, tricyclics lose the ability to antagonize the D_2 receptor (characteristic of phenothiazines) but retain affinity to interact with many other receptor types. Their primary initial effect appears to be the *blockade of reuptake mechanisms* for biogenic monoamines. Tricyclics also can *block receptors* (muscarinic, serotonergic, histaminic, and α-adrenoceptors) but this may be unrelated to their therapeutic benefits.

Imipramine, amitriptyline and doxepin are serotonin reuptake blockers and have prominent sedative effects. Their major metabolites, desipramine and nortriptyline, are better blockers of norepinephrine reuptake and have less sedative effects. Although reuptake blockade occurs immediately, several weeks must elapse before the antidepressant action is exerted. The antidepressant action may relate to modification in receptor regulation (down regulation of receptors). Adverse effects occur from receptor blockade at the initiation of medication, the most troublesome of which is orthostatic hypotension and delayed cardiac conduction. Accidental and deliberate overdose in patients occurs frequently and constitutes a serious medical emergency. Major symptoms of overdose include: coma with shock, respiratory depression, agitation, seizures, hyperpyrexia, bowel and bladder paralysis, and various cardiac manifestations.

Imipramine and amitriptyline also have several other therapeutic uses including neurogenic pain, phobias, panic, cataplexy, and bruxism. They also are useful as secondary drugs in enuresis, eating and attention deficit disorders.

2. SECOND GENERATION DRUGS

These drugs were developed in attempts to eliminate some of the troublesome side effect, i.e., cardiac manifestations and orthostatic hypotension, and secondarily to reduce some of the drowsiness and weight gain which also occurred with the tricyclics.

a. Fluoxetine, sertraline and paroxetine are selective inhibitors of serotonin reuptake. They are used extensively to treat nondelusional moderately depressed patients.
b. Trazodone is also a weak inhibitor of serotonin reuptake. It is an unpredictable drug in that some patients show marked improvement, others no effect. An initial drug trial is given primarily to patients who are intolerant to the adverse anticholinergic effects of the other drugs. It has major sedative effects and infrequently causes priapism.
c. Maprotiline is not a selective reuptake inhibitor. It used for manic-depressive illness of the depressed type and for depressed neurosis. It will evoke seizures on high or rapidly escalating doses.

3. MONOAMINE OXIDASE (MAO) INHIBITORS

Phenelzine is the drug of choice for atypical depression. Optimal antidepressant activity is achieved when there is 60-80% inhibition of monoamine oxidase (as measured in platelets). The most serious adverse effect of MAO inhibitors is hypertensive crisis, which may occur within hours of ingestion of contraindicated substances (tyramine from cheese. etc.); prodromal signs may include palpitations or frequent headaches. Hypertensive crisis is characterized by headache, palpitation, neck stiffness or soreness, nausea, vomiting, sweating (sometimes with fever or cold, clammy skin), photophobia, tachycardia or bradycardia, constricting chest pain, and dilated pupils. Potentially fatal intracranial bleeding may result from this crisis.

4. CONVULSIVE THERAPY

Electroconvulsive therapy (or a convulsant drug, Flurothyl) is used as alternatives for treatment of depression if the patient does not respond to drug therapy.

5. LITHIUM

Lithium is the preferred drug for treating bipolar affective (manic-depressive) disorder. Because of its slow onset of action, concurrent use of an antipsychotic is required in the severely manic patient until the mania is controlled. Lithium interferes with the phosphoinositol cycle by blocking the second messenger metabolic cascade at the monophosphatase level. High correlation exists between plasma concentrations and therapeutic efficacy and toxicity. Dietary sodium should remain at a constant intake.
Adverse effects include: tremor, muscle hyperirritability, aphasia, and mental confusion. Rare, chronic toxicities include goitrogenic hypothyrodism, renal tubular necrosis, and diabetes insipidus.

C. OBSESSIVE-COMPULSIVE DISORDER

Clomipramine is the drug of choice and it will improve significantly 50-70% of the patients. Responses to drug therapy has a slow onset of action, taking up to 10 weeks for full response. For intractable cases, surgical cingulotomy is performed.

D. ANTIPSYCHOTICS

Antipsychotic drugs ameliorate the symptoms of psychosis including schizophrenia, acute mania, schizoaffective disorders,and borderline personality disorders. In addition, these agents are used as antiemetics and for a variety of other disorders such as chronic multiple tics, neurogenic pain, Huntington's Disease, ballismus, infantile autism, intractable hiccups and some symptoms of conduct and behavioral disorders.

1. Phenothiazine antipsychotics are divided into three chemical classes based on side chain:
   a. Perphenazine and fluphenazine (piperazine chain): The most potent as antipsychotics and antiemetics but have the highest incidence of extrapyramidal side effects.
   b. Chlorpromazine (aliphatic chain): These agents have both antipsychotic and antiemetic efficacy but adverse effects have made them obsolete in treating schizophrenia. Chlorpromazine remains the drug of choice for intractable hiccups.
   c. Thioridazine (piperidine chain): These are the least potent agents as antipsychotics and have lowest incidence of extrapyramidal adverse effects.

They are not used as antiemetics; patients on thioridazine should be monitored for retinopathy.

2. <u>Haloperidol</u> is used extensively, in particular for initial stabilization of the psychotic patient. It causes fewer adverse autonomic effects than phenothiazines, however, the induction of tardive dyskinesia and other extrapyramidal adverse effects limits its chronic use.

3. Other antipsychotic drugs include:
   a. <u>Thiothixene</u>: The drug of choice for borderline personality disorders.
   b. <u>Pimozide</u>: The major clinical use for this drug to prevent acute exacerbation of chronic schizophrenia and to suppress motor and vocal tics in Tourette's disorder.
   c. <u>Loxapine</u>: This drug is indicated for the treatment of schizoaffective disorders because its major metabolite <u>amoxapine</u> is an antidepressant.
   d. <u>Clozapine</u>: This drug lacks extrapyramidal adverse effects and is indicated for patients who are severely disturbed, are refractory to other treatment, have tardive dyskinesia and those who are unusually sensitive to extrapyramidal adverse effects. Patients on this drug must be monitored weekly for agranulocytosis.

The adverse effects of antipsychotic drugs correlate to their affinity to different receptors. As D_2 *dopamine receptor antagonists* they cause extrapyramidal effects: (1) Parkinson's syndrome; (2) perioral tremor, a late variant of parkinsonism; (3) akathisia, (4) acute dystonia; (5) malignant neuroleptic syndrome and (6) tardive dyskinesia. As *dopamine antagonists* in the *tubero-infundibular pathway*, the antipsychotic drugs cause hyperprolactinemia which can result in amenorrhea, galactorrhea, infertility and impotence. Sedation occurs from affinity to and *blockade of the histamine H_1 receptor*. Orthostatic hypotension, impotence, and failure to ejaculate, are adverse effects mediated through *α-adrenoceptor blockade*. Anticholinergic effects, including a toxic-confusional state at high doses, are mediated by *muscarinic cholinoceptor blockade*. Weight gain is common with antipsychotic drugs and requires monitoring of food intake.

D. DRUGS OF ABUSE

1. <u>Drug abuse</u> refers to the use, usually by self administration, of any drug in a manner that deviates from the approved medical or social patterns within a culture. <u>Drug misuse</u> is an inappropriate use of the drug. Social costs per year for drug dependence is estimated to be 60 billion for illicit drugs, 120 billion for alcohol and 65 billion for nicotine.

2. On the basis of commonality of characteristics and the phenomena of cross-tolerance and cross-dependence the major drugs of abuse can be placed into seven categories. Cross-tolerance and cross-dependence only occurs within a class.

    a. Opioids
    b. Sedative - hypnotics, including alcohol
    c. Stimulants - caffeine, amphetamine, cocaine
    d. Hallucinogens
       1) Psychedelic - LSD, psilocybin, mescaline
       2) Deliriant - Phencyclidine, anticholinergics
    e. Cannabis - marihuana
    f. Tobacco - nicotine
    g. Inhalants - nitrous oxide, gasoline, volatile solvents, aerosols

3. Physical dependence is defined by a withdrawal syndrome, which for a first approximation, is a rebound in the drug responses with a time course set by the declining blood levels. A prolonged secondary phase can occur. Of the seven classes, physical dependence is greater than psychological dependence for only the opioids and sedative-hypnotics including alcohol. Tolerance for the drugs of abuse is primarily a change in cellular dynamics rather than kinetics with opioids and amphetamines exhibiting marked tolerance.

4. Detoxification is the same for all drugs that produce physical dependence. This involves substituting a longer-acting, orally effective, pharmacologically equivalent drug for the abused drug. The patient is stabilized on the substitute and then it is gradually withdrawn. There is a high recidivism rate among drug abusers. Currently there are many psychotherapeutic programs after detoxification, but these programs have success rates varying from 10% to perhaps a maximum of 50%.

5. Opioid intoxication effects on performance includes mental clouding, faulty judgement and reduced ability to concentrate. Physical signs of abuse include pupillary constriction, depression and apathy.

   Withdrawal from morphine, heroin, codeine produced peak abstinence symptoms at 36-72 hours (for meperidine, 7-12 hours and methadone, about 7 days). Early symptoms at 10-12 hours include: rhinorrhea, perspiration, lacrimation and yawning. Intermediate symptoms at 18-24 hours: mydriasis, piloerection, anorexia, muscular tremors. Peak symptoms at 36-72 hours: restlessness, hot flashes alternating with chills, increase in blood pressure and heart rate, increases in rate and depth of respiration, fever of 1° or more, nausea, retching, vomiting and diarrhea. Withdrawal from an opioid is generally not life threatening although almost unbearable.

6. Sedative-hypnotics, including alcohol: Performance decrements occur at low levels. For example, "fitness for duty" laws have established blood alcohol level of 0.04% where prior experience can not compensate for the drug induced performance degradation. Withdrawal includes a progression of symptoms varying from tremulousness to convulsions and toxic psychosis. Withdrawal from these drugs can be life-threatening.

7. Stimulants: Low doses produce wakefulness, and in sleep deprived individuals, they reduce fatigue and return capability to perform psychomotor tasks to baseline levels. Perception of heightened performance is only a perception and not a reality. With complex tasks there is a decrement in performance. Adverse effects to high doses induce paranoid ideation, hallucinations, depression and more rarely seizure activity and cardiac arrhythmias. For amphetamines after prolonged self-administration (a "run"), prolonged sleep, apathy and depression are common. *Marked tolerance* develops to the *amphetamines* but not to cocaine or to caffeine.

8. The psychedelic hallucinogens - LSD, psilocybin, and mescaline: Differ primarily in potency; synesthesias and "flashbacks" are unique features.

9. The deliriant hallucinogens - phencyclidine: Intoxication at low doses resembles an acute confused state; at higher doses, serious neurological, cardiovascular, and psychotic reactions occur.

10. Cannabis - marihuana: Casual users have performance decrements not seen in chronic users. However, chronic users show hostility and personality problems not seen in the casual user. The "amotivational syndrome" associated with chronic heavy users may not be specific but is a general syndrome seen in chronic users of psychoactive drugs, primarily those in the sedative-hypnotic class.

11. Tobacco-nicotine: Nicotine causes an alerting pattern in the EEG; also it decreases skeletal muscle tone, appetite and irritability; and has a mild euphorigenic effect. Withdrawal is variable but increased appetite and inability to concentrate may persist for months.

12. Inhalants: Acute toxicity to the aerosol propellants and volatile solvents is respiratory arrest and cardiac arrhythmias. Direct administration of the aerosol propellants has resulted in laryngospasm, airway freezing and suffocation due to an occluded airway. Chronic toxicity varies, depending on the solvent, but is characterized by tissue damage, which probably is the reason the solvent abusers are the most difficult group to rehabilitate.

REVIEW QUESTIONS

ONE BEST ANSWER

1. Opioids therapeutically are used as all of the following **EXCEPT**:

   A. Analgesics
   B. Anti-tussives
   C. Sedatives
   D. Anti-diarrheals

2. All of the following statements regarding opioid analgesics are correct **EXCEPT**:

   A. Sharp, stabbing pain is better relieved by opioids than severe, dull, constant pain.
   B. Cough suppression can be obtained at lower doses than needed for analgesia.
   C. Pain relief provided by opioids increases with age.
   D. The treatment of pain with opioids is symptomatic treatment only.

3. Naloxone:

   A. Has a low affinity for mu receptors.
   B. Is effective only by the intravenous route.
   C. Acts by non-competitive inhibition.
   D. Will worsen the respiratory depression caused by barbiturates.
   E. Has a significantly longer half-life than morphine.

4. Tolerance develops to all of the following opioid effects **EXCEPT**:

   A. Analgesia
   B. Miosis
   C. Sedation
   D. Respiratory depression
   E. Cough suppression

5. The Minimum Alveolar Concentration (MAC) is:

   A. The alveolar concentration at which 100% of the patients fail to respond to standard surgical stimuli.
   B. The alveolar concentration which is lethal for 50% of the patients.
   C. The alveolar concentration at which 50% of the patients fail to respond to standard surgical stimuli.
   D. The alveolar concentration at which 50% of the administered anesthetic is dissolved in the blood.

6. All of the following statements about pain pathways are correct **EXCEPT**:

   A. Primary afferent fibers carrying information about painful stimuli synapse in the spinal cord dorsal horn in the substantia gelatinosa.
   B. Painful information is conveyed from the periphery to the central nervous system via A-delta and C-fibers.
   C. Local anesthetics reversibly block nerve conduction.
   D. Opioids prevent the initiation of pain impulses.
   E. Bradykinin is an initiator of pain impulses.

7. All of the following statements are true regarding nitrous oxide **EXCEPT**:

   A. Nitrous oxide is a good analgesic agent.
   B. Long term exposure to trace concentrations of nitrous oxide may cause pernicious anemia.
   C. Nitrous oxide is an incomplete anesthetic.
   D. Nitrous oxide has a slow induction rate.
   E. Nitrous oxide is relatively insoluble in the blood.

113

ONE BEST ANSWER

8. All of the following statements regarding endogenous opioids are true **EXCEPT**:

   A. Administration of an opioid antagonist does not lower the pain threshold in humans.
   B. Enkephalins are found in the brain and spinal cord.
   C. Endorphins coexist with ACTH in pituitary secretory granules.
   D. Pro-opiomelanocortin gives rise to met- and leu-enkephalin.
   E. Endogenous opioids may mediate the analgesic effects of acupuncture and placebo administration.

9. An ideal anesthetic is one that produces:

   A. Muscle relaxation
   B. Analgesia
   C. Unconsciousness
   D. All of the above

10. Local anesthetics block:

   A. The initiation of pain impulses in the periphery.
   B. The release of neurotransmitters from primary afferents in the spinal cord.
   C. The propagation of pain impulses along axons.
   D. The processing of painful information in the thalamus.

11. General anesthesia with:

   A. Enflurane produces fluoride toxicity.
   B. Halothane produces a dose-dependent hypotension.
   C. Thiopental produces myocardial stimulation.
   D. Nitrous oxide produces hallucinations following recovery.

12. The "second gas" effect most commonly is seen with:

   A. Ketamine
   B. Halothane
   C. Methoxyflurane
   D. Nitrous Oxide
   E. Diazepam

13. All of the following statements concerning general anesthesia are correct **EXCEPT**:

   A. Inhalation anesthetics have low therapeutic indices.
   B. General anesthetics produce their effects by acting at specific receptor sites.
   C. The lipid solubility of anesthetic compounds is an important determinant for anesthetic potency.
   D. Synaptic transmission is more susceptible to general anesthetics than axonal transmission.

14. Which of the following agents functionally is classified as a mixed opioid agonist/antagonist?

   A. Propoxyphene
   B. Naltrexone
   C. Pentazocine
   D. Fentanyl
   E. Meperidine

15. All of the following opioid effects are central nervous system effects **EXCEPT**:

   A. Respiratory depression
   B. Truncal rigidity
   C. Nausea and vomiting
   D. Postoperative urinary retention
   E. Miosis

16. Which of the following factors influence the rate of induction of inhalation anesthetics?

   A. Blood flow
   B. Blood solubility
   C. Cardiac output
   D. Ventilation rate
   E. All of the above

17. The drug of choice to treat malignant hyperthermia is:

   A. Propranolol
   B. Dantrolene
   C. Diazepam
   D. Piroxicam
   E. Valproate

114

18. Which of the following agents produces a high incidence of phlebitis?

    A. Ketamine
    B. Thiopental
    C. Diazepam
    D. Methoxyflurane
    E. Halothane

19. Which of the following general anesthetic agents sensitizes the myocardium to adrenergic agonists and may increase the likelihood of arrhythmias?

    A. Halothane
    B. Nitrous Oxide
    C. Thiopental
    D. Ketamine
    E. Diazepam

20. Vasoconstrictors often are added to local anesthetics to:

    A. Increase systemic absorption.
    B. Prolong the duration of action.
    C. Minimize bradycardia.
    D. Prevent hypotension.

21. Which of the following local anesthetic agents can be used for topical application **only**?

    A. Lidocaine
    B. Procaine
    C. Mepivacaine
    D. Benzocaine

22. Adverse effects which can result from the administration of an opioid analgesic include all of the following **EXCEPT**:

    A. Urinary retention
    B. Nausea and vomiting
    C. Diarrhea
    D. Dysphoria
    E. Constriction of bronchiolar smooth muscle

23. Signs and symptoms of CNS toxicity caused by local anesthetics include: dizziness, numbness, and visual and auditory disturbances. The most probable cause of the toxicity is:

    A. Patient hypersensitivity to the anesthetic agent.
    B. Excessive blood levels of the anesthetic agent.
    C. Patient hypersensitivity to the vasoconstrictor.
    D. Psychogenic causes.
    E. Deterioration of the anesthetic agent.

24. Analgesic efficacy is greatest for:

    A. Aspirin
    B. Codeine
    C. Aspirin + Acetaminophen
    D. Acetaminophen
    E. Codeine + Aspirin

25. Tonic/clonic muscle activity and seizures have been associated with:

    A. Halothane
    B. Enflurane
    C. Methoxyflurane
    D. Ketamine

26. Properties associated with the mu receptor include:

    A. Sedation
    B. Analgesia
    C. Respiratory depression
    D. Physical dependence
    E. All of the above

27. Opioid antagonists can reverse most of the effects produced by opioids **EXCEPT**:

    A. Respiratory depression
    B. Analgesia
    C. Sedation
    D. Miosis
    E. Anti-tussive effect

115

ONE BEST ANSWER

28. Among the hallucinogens, psilocybin, mescaline and LSD, one might expect them to differ in which one of the following characteristics?

A. Development of tolerance
B. Development of cross tolerance
C. Potency
D. Nature of the hallucinations
E. Psychological effects

29. Benzodiazepines and phenothiazines share which effect?

A. Physical dependence
B. Sedation
C. Extrapyramidal symptoms
D. Antiemetic action
E. Muscle-relaxant activity

30. Which one of the following is the predominant process responsible for terminating the central depressant action of a single dose of pentobarbital?

A. Metabolic degradation
B. Renal excretion
C. Physical redistribution
D. Reuptake at the synapse
E. None of the above

31. Degeneration of the nasal septum is most often associated with abuse of:

A. LSD
B. Ethyl alcohol
C. Amphetamine
D. Cocaine

32. Which one of the following compounds produces Parkinsonism?

A. Amphetamine
B. Ecstasy (MDMA)
C. DMT (Dimethyltryptamine)
D. MPTP (Methylphenyltetrahydropyridine)

33. Acute intermittent porphyria is a contraindication for most sedative-hypnotic drugs because they:

A. Induce one form of cytochrome P-450
B. Increase the rate of synthesis of the Y protein (Ligandins)
C. Inhibit porphobilinogen deaminase
D. Induce aminolevulinic acid (ALA) synthetase

34. The preferred drug for attention deficit disorder in children is:

A. Theophylline
B. Methylphenidate
C. Diazepam
D. Dextroamphetamine

35. Antipsychotic effects of phenothiazines are thought to be caused by the blockade of which receptor system?

A. Limbic serotonin
B. Striatal dopamine
C. Striatal enkephalin
D. Limbic dopamine

36. Trihexyphenidyl is the drug of choice for treating which one of the following primary symptoms of Parkinson's disease?

A. Rigidity
B. Bradykinesia
C. Postural instability
D. Resting tremor

37. Bromocriptine is:

A. A peripheral decarboxylase inhibitor
B. A dopamine receptor agonist
C. A dopamine releaser
D. Monoamine oxidase B inhibitor

116

ONE BEST ANSWER

38. Triazolam and alprazolam have shorter half-lives than other benzodiazepines because:

   A. They have a hydroxy group which is conjugated
   B. They have an extra ring that prevents metabolism to a nordiazepam analogue
   C. They have higher lipid solubility so that redistribution is faster
   D. They are more water soluble and can be excreted in the urine unchanged

39. The principle cause for pathologic changes in the nervous system with alcoholism is considered to be:

   A. Direct toxicity of ethanol
   B. Direct toxicity of acetaldehyde
   C. Inflammatory effects of alcohol
   D. Malnutrition

40. In a patient with renal impairment a prolonged duration of action would occur most likely for which one of the following sedative-hypnotics?

   A. Pentobarbital
   B. Diazepam
   C. Thiopental
   D. Phenobarbital
   E. Alprazolam

41. During the establishment of an adequate daily phenytoin dose, small increases in dose are often required in the therapeutic range. The primary pharmacological reason is:

   A. Poor oral absorption of phenytoin
   B. A change in extent of protein binding
   C. Saturation of the enzyme involved in phenytoin metabolism
   D. An alteration in the affinity of the phenytoin receptor

42. The therapeutic use of diazepam in epilepsy is associated with which disorder?

   A. Generalized tonic-clonic seizures
   B. Absences
   C. Partial seizures with complex symptomatology
   D. Febrile seizures
   E. Status epilepticus

43. Ballismus is controlled with which one of the following drugs?

   A. Selegiline
   B. Benztropine
   C. Haloperidol
   D. Carbamazepine
   E. L-DOPA

44. Surgery is performed if medical management is inadequate in which one of the following forms of seizures?

   A. Simple partial seizures (Jacksonian)
   B. Complex partial seizures (temporal lobe)
   C. Clonic-tonic-clonic seizures
   D. Tonic seizures
   E. Clonic seizures of juvenile onset

45. The extrapyramidal adverse effects of antipsychotic drugs include all of the following **EXCEPT**:

   A. Akathisia
   B. Acute dystonias
   C. Myoclonus
   D. Tardive dyskinesia

46. All of the following phenothiazines are used for their antiemetic action **EXCEPT**:

   A. Prochlorperazine
   B. Promethazine
   C. Fluphenazine
   D. Thioridazine

ONE BEST ANSWER

47. Lithium is characterized by all of the following **EXCEPT**:

   A. Interferes with the phosphoinositol cycle
   B. Is indicated in recurrent endogenous depressions with a cyclic pattern
   C. Good correlations exist between plasma concentrations and therapeutic efficacy and toxicity
   D. Causes renal tubular necrosis and diabetes insipidus in a high percentage of lithium-treated patients

48. Withdrawal from a sedative-hypnotic can include all of the following **EXCEPT**:

   A. Tonic-clonic seizures
   B. Toxic psychosis
   C. Somnolence
   D. Cardiovascular collapse

49. Withdrawal signs may occur after cessation of chronic use of all of the following **EXCEPT**:

   A. Meperidine
   B. Marihuana
   C. Alcohol
   D. Secobarbital

50. All of the following apply to the phenomenon of tolerance to opioid analgesics **EXCEPT**:

   A. Tolerance develops faster with large doses given at short intervals, than with small doses given at longer intervals
   B. Tolerance develops at different rates for the various responses to opioid analgesics
   C. An individual tolerant to morphine will also be tolerant to meperidine and methadone
   D. Once acquired, tolerance is lost only after several weeks of drug abstinence

51. All of the following drugs are useful for muscle relaxation due to an acute injury **EXCEPT**:

   A. Phenobarbital
   B. Cyclobenzaprine
   C. Diazepam
   D. Buspirone

52. A peripheral decarboxylase inhibitor, such as carbidopa, is administered with L-DOPA because of all of the following reasons **EXCEPT**:

   A. Abnormal involuntary movements and personality disorders are reduced
   B. The effective oral dose of L-DOPA can be reduced
   C. The incidence of nausea and vomiting is markedly decreased
   D. The risk for cardiac arrhythmias and further hypotension is decreased

53. In manganese toxicity there is a DECREASE in striatal dopamine levels; rational therapy could include treatment with all of the following drugs **EXCEPT**:

   A. Anticholinergic drug
   B. Bromocriptine
   C. Haloperidol
   D. L-DOPA

54. Valproate indications include all of the following **EXCEPT**:

   A. Atypical absence
   B. Tonic-clonic seizures
   C. Atonic/Akinetic seizures
   E. Infantile spasms

55. The drug of choice for treating obsessive-compulsive disorders is which one of the following drugs?

   A. Clomipramine
   B. Imipramine
   C. Perphenazine
   D. Diazepam

56. When thiopental is used as an induction agent, the onset of anesthesia is determined by all of the following **EXCEPT**:

   A. The creation of a gradient by i.v. injection
   B. The high blood flow to the brain relative to other tissues
   C. Its rapid penetration into the brain from the blood (high lipid solubility)
   D. Its redistribution from brain into muscle and fat

ONE BEST ANSWER

57. Early symptoms of opioid analgesic withdrawal includes all of the following **EXCEPT**:

    A. Rhinorrhea
    B. Diarrhea
    C. Perspiration
    D. Lacrimation

58. Transient symptoms of tachycardia and hypertension experienced as a result of alcohol consumption is probably best explained by:

    A. Release of epinephrine from the adrenal gland
    B. Release of vasopressin from the posterior pituitary
    C. Direct effects of alcohol on the heart and vascular smooth muscles
    D. Effects of acetaldehyde on the heart and vascular smooth muscles

59. Alcohol may be eliminated by metabolism, excretion into the urine or other body fluids, or expired in the process of breathing. About what per cent of the alcohol ingested is metabolized?

    A. 10-20%
    B. 30-40%
    C. 50-60%
    D. 70-80%
    E. 90-95%

MATCHING: Questions 60-72.

A. Amantadine   K. Estazolam   U. Midazolam
B. Baclofen   L. Flumazenil   V. Quazepam
C. Buprenorphine   M. Fluoxetine   W. Phencyclidine
D. Bupropion   N. Fluorothyl   X. Pimozide
E. Buspirone   O. Heroin   Y. Procyclidine
F. Carbamazepine   P. Isoflurane   Z. Selegiline
G. Clozapine   Q. Loxapine
H. Cyclobenzaprine R. LSD
I. Doxepin   S. Maprotiline
J. Dantrolene   T. Marihuana

60. Drug of choice for both rapidly cycling manic-depressive episodes and trigeminal neuralgia

61. Benzodiazepine antagonist

62. An drug that will slow the progression of the Parkinson's disease.

63. Drug causes distortion in sensory perception, especially vision; synesthesias, and "flashbacks" may occur

64. Second generation antipsychotic which can be used in patients with tardive dyskinesia but must monitor for agranulocytosis

65. Common symptoms of use include reddening of the conjunctiva and an "amotivational syndrome" can be expressed

66. Convulsive agent used in treating endogenous or severe reactive depression

67. Drug of choice for conscious sedation.

68. Antipsychotic drug whose use is limited to preventing acute exacerbation of chronic schizophrenia and to suppress the motor and vocal tics in Tourette's disorder.

69. In moderately severe intoxication, patient "zombie-like" but combative and hostile.

70. An antidyskinetic used when rigidity is the presenting symptom of Parkinson's disease.

71. Antipsychotic drug which is used in schizoaffective disorders, partially because its antidepressant metabolite, amoxapine, reaches therapeutic blood levels.

72. Second generation antidepressant that was withdrawn and reintroduced after the seizure incidence was defined.

73. Second generation antidepressant that is indicated for manic-depressive illness of the depressed type and for depressive neurosis.

74. A CNS skeletal muscle relaxant that has efficacy for acute but not chronic muscle spasms.

MATCHING

The adverse effects of the antipsychotic and antidepressant drugs are associated with their capability to antagonize various receptors. Match the receptor type to the adverse effects.

      A. Histamine - H_1
      B. Alpha-1-Adrenergic
      C. Muscarinic
      D. Dopamine D_2

75. Postural hypotension, reflex tachycardia

76. Blurred vision, urinary retention, memory dysfunction

77. Galactorrhea, akathisia

CHAPTER 7: <u>AUTACOIDS AND THE THERAPY OF INFLAMMATION</u>

I. **AUTACOIDS**

A. HISTAMINE AND ANTIHISTAMINES

1. HISTAMINE
   a. General Considerations
      1) <u>Tissue Localization</u>: stored in the blood in basophils; stored in tissues in mast cells; high concentrations in the skin, mucosa of the bronchi, and intestinal mucosa; also found in CNS neurons
      2) <u>Synthesis</u>: synthesized from histidine by L-histidine decarboxylase
      3) <u>Metabolism</u>: two main pathways; metabolites excreted in the urine
         a) Ring methylation -- catalyzed by histamine-N-methyltransferase; further metabolized by monoamine oxidase
         b) Oxidative deamination -- catalyzed by diamine oxidase
      4) <u>Tissue Release</u>: release and production stimulated by damage to cells and tissue; antigen-antibody reactions, snake venoms and drugs (e.g., curare and morphine) also can liberate histamine from tissue stores
      5) <u>Functions</u>: involved in hypersensitivity reactions, regulation of gastric secretions, and CNS neurotransmission
   b. Receptor Types:
      1) H_1 -- mediate bronchoconstriction, contraction of the gut and vascular dilation
      2) H_2 -- mediate gastric secretion and vascular dilation
      3) H_3 -- localized in both the peripheral and central nervous system; mediate synthesis and release of histamine from non-mast cell sites
   c. Pharmacologic Effects
      1) <u>Cardiovascular System</u>: dilation of small blood vessels results in flushing and decreased systemic pressure; increased capillary permeability results in edema; effects are mediated by both H_1 and H_2 receptors
         a) **Triple Response:** intradermally injected histamine elicits: 1) a localized red spot, 2) a brighter red flush or flare extending about 1 cm beyond the original red spot, and 3) a wheal that develops in 1-2 minutes
      2) <u>Smooth Muscle</u>: with the exception of vascular smooth muscle (which is relaxed), most other smooth muscle is stimulated by histamine. Constrictor effects (H_1) are most prominent in the bronchi and uterus; responses of intestinal muscle vary, and there are few effects on the bladder, gallbladder, ureter and iris
      3) <u>Glands</u>: stimulates secretions from the salivary, bronchial and gastric glands; effects mediated by H_2 receptors
      4) <u>Nerve Endings</u>: stimulates nerve endings causing pain and itching; mediated by H_1 receptors

    d. Toxicity
       1) Life-threatening symptoms include shock (general vasodilation and a marked fall in blood pressure) and severe bronchoconstriction. Mediators other than histamine also are involved in the anaphylactic response.
       2) Most effective treatment for anaphylactoid reactions is epinephrine; antihistamines and glucocorticoids decrease the magnitude of the late occurring response (e.g., hives and itching).
    e. Clinical Uses
       1) Used diagnostically for: achlorhydria (inability of histamine to induce gastric secretions) and pheochromocytoma (histamine-induced release of adrenal catecholamines)
       2) Betazole: H_2 agonist used to test for gastric acid-secreting ability

2. H_1 ANTIHISTAMINES
    a. Possess sedative, local anesthetic and anticholinergic properties.
    b. Modify some of the signs and symptoms of histamine release, but do **NOT** prevent the release of histamine from mast cells.
    c. Pharmacologic Effects
       1) Smooth Muscle: antagonize the constrictor action of histamine on respiratory and vascular smooth muscle; antagonize the changes in capillary permeability produced by histamine that result in edema
       2) CNS: bind to H_1 receptors in the CNS; can cause both depression and stimulation; depression commonly occurs with older agents causing sedation; stimulation of receptors may cause restlessness, nervousness and insomnia; may possess antiemetic effects and be effective against motion sickness
       3) Autonomic Nervous System: many antihistamines possess anticholinergic properties
       4) Local Anesthetic Effect: some antihistamines have local anesthetic and quinidine-like properties
    d. Absorption, Metabolism and Excretion
       1) Well absorbed following oral administration
       2) Widely distributed and extensively metabolized; induce hepatic microsomal enzymes; may facilitate their own metabolism; frequently eliminated more rapidly by children
       3) Metabolites eliminated in the urine
    e. Side Effects
       1) Sedation: most common; may limit use
       2) Gastric effects: loss of appetite, constipation or diarrhea, nausea and vomiting
       3) Anticholinergic effects: dry mouth, cough, palpitations, headache
       4) Allergic dermatitis with topical application
    f. Toxicity
       1) Initial central excitatory effects: hallucinations, excitement, ataxia, convulsions, etc.

2) Terminally there is coma, respiratory collapse and death within 2-18 hrs; treatment is supportive.

g. Therapeutic Uses and Selected Agents

  1) **Allergy**: used to relieve itching, edema and allergic rhinitis; some of these agents also are promoted as OTC sedative drugs

    a) <u>First Generation Antihistamines</u>

      (1) Significant sedative, anticholinergic and antiemetic effects
         Diphenhydramine
         Promethazine
         Clemastine

      (2) Fewer sedative and anticholinergic effects
         Tripelennamine
         Chlorpheniramine

    b) <u>Second Generation Antihistamines</u> -- little or no sedation, anticholinergic activity or antiemetic effects

      (1) Reported to interact with inhibitors of drug metabolism to promote arrhythmias; contraindicated in persons with severe hepatic disease
         Terfenadine
         Astemizole

      (2) No reported drug interactions
         Loratidine

  2) **Motion Sickness, Vertigo and Emesis**

    a) Dimenhydrinate
    b) Meclizine
    c) Prochlorperazine
    d) Promethazine

3. H_2 ANTIHISTAMINES

a. Competitive antagonists at the H_2 receptor

b. Inhibit gastric secretions elicited by histamine

c. Well absorbed orally; eliminated in the urine

d. Specific Agents

  1) <u>Cimetidine</u>: prescribed for treatment of duodenal and gastric ulcers; side effects include: diarrhea, nausea and vomiting, myalgia, skin rashes, loss of libido, impotence, gynecomastia; inhibits cytochrome P450 and may potentiate other drugs

  2) <u>Ranitidine</u>: increased potency and longer duration of action; does not inhibit cytochrome P450; no antiandrogenic effects

  3) <u>Famotidine</u>

  4) <u>Nizatidine</u>

4. INHIBITORS OF AUTACOID RELEASE (HISTAMINE AND LEUKOTRIENES) FROM MAST CELLS

a. Available agents are cromolyn sodium and nedocromil sodium

b. Used prophylactically for asthma and seasonal allergic rhinitis

B. SEROTONIN AND SEROTONIN ANTAGONISTS

1. SEROTONIN (5-HYDROXYTRYPTAMINE, 5-HT)
   a. General Considerations
      1) <u>Tissue Localization</u>: high concentrations in platelets, enterochromaffin cells in gastrointestinal tract, and in the CNS
      2) <u>Synthesis</u>: synthesized from tryptophan; rate-limiting enzyme is tryptophan-5-hydroxylase; taken up into secretory granules and stored
      3) <u>Metabolism</u>: oxidative deamination by monoamine oxidase and aldehyde dehydrogenase to form 5-hydroxyindoleacetic acid (5- HIAA); metabolites are excreted in the urine
      4) <u>Functions</u>: may play a role in hemostasis and certain vasospastic diseases; regulation of gastrointestinal motility; CNS neurotransmission
   b. Receptor Types
      1) $5\text{-}HT_1$
      2) $5\text{-}HT_2$
      3) $5\text{-}HT_3$
   c. Pharmacologic Effects
      1) <u>Cardiovascular System</u>: primary effect is vasoconstriction ($5\text{-}HT_2/5\text{-}HT_1$) of most arteries, veins and venules; effects of other contractile agonists (NE, histamine and angiotensin II) are amplified; vasodilation ($5\text{-}HT_1$) of small vessels in skeletal muscle; increased blood pressure; positive inotropic and chronotropic effects on the heart ($5\text{-}HT_1$)
      2) <u>Respiratory System</u>: increased respiratory rate
      3) <u>Smooth Muscle</u>: increased motility of the small intestine; contraction of uterine and bronchial smooth muscle.
      4) <u>Nerve Endings</u>: stimulation or inhibition of nerve endings; $5\text{-}HT_3$ receptors on sensory nerves may mediate the ability of 5-HT to cause pain and itching.
      5) <u>Carcinoid Syndrome</u>: tumors release 5-HT, bradykinin, epinephrine and histamine to produce: 1) flushing, 2) wide swings in blood pressure, 3) colic and 4) bronchiolar constriction.
2. SEROTONIN ANTAGONISTS
   a. Specific Agents
      1) <u>Ketanserin</u>: blocks $5\text{-}HT_2$ receptors; affinity also for α_1, H_1 and dopamine receptors; under investigation in clinical trials in the U.S. for use in diseases where excessive vascular tone may be caused by 5-HT release from platelets (e.g., Raynaud's syndrome); lowers blood pressure in man
      2) <u>Methysergide</u>: congener of LSD; inhibits the vasoconstrictor and pressor effects of 5-HT; used for treatment of carcinoid syndrome and the prophylactic treatment of migraines
      3) <u>Cyproheptadine</u>: potent antihistamine and antiserotonin agent; used to treat pruritic dermatoses and carcinoid syndrome

C. BRADYKININ
1. GENERAL CONSIDERATIONS
   a. Bradykinin exists in the plasma in an inactive form.
   b. It is formed from the $\alpha 2$ globulin precursor, bradykininogen, by the plasma enzyme kallikrein.
   c. Bradykinin has a half-life of about 15 seconds; a single passage through the pulmonary vascular bed destroys 80-90% of the kinins; the principal catabolizing enzymes in the lung are kininase I (carboxypeptidase) and kininase II (angiotensin converting enzyme).
   d. Functions
      1) Pain: bradykinin receptors are localized in the CNS in sites involved in nociception; it produces pain in experimental models and in humans
      2) Inflammation: kinins mimic the manifestations of inflammation; they may be involved in rhinitis, gout, endotoxic shock and disseminated intravascular coagulation
      3) Renal Function and Blood Pressure: bradykinin may be involved in the local regulation of renal function; the kinin system may be activated to blunt the effects of pressor agents
1. RECEPTOR TYPES
   a. B_1 -- synthesis induced by trauma or pathological conditions
   b. B_2 -- mediate the majority of bradykinin effects including: vasodilation, pain, smooth muscle contraction and increased capillary permeability
   c. B_3 -- may be involved in smooth muscle contraction in the gastrointestinal tract.
3. PHARMACOLOGIC EFFECTS
   a. Cardiovascular System: potent vasodilator (10X more potent than histamine) of blood vessels in the muscle, kidney, viscera, heart and brain; if administered intravenously the kinins cause flushing, headache and decreased systemic pressure; reflex increase in heart rate and cardiac output; plasma kinins increase capillary permeability which leads to edema
   b. Smooth Muscle: potent constrictor of uterine, bronchiolar, and gastrointestinal smooth muscle
   c. Nerve Endings: potent algesic agent
4. BRADYKININ ANTAGONISTS AND KALLIKREIN INHIBITORS
   Currently being developed; initial trials suggest that they may be useful in the treatment of cold symptoms caused by rhinovirus, burn pain and allergic asthma.

D. ANGIOTENSIN

1. GENERAL CONSIDERATIONS
   a. Synthesis: The enzyme renin, acts on angiotensinogen to form angiotensin I; in the lung (primarily), angiotensin I is converted to angiotensin II by dipeptide hydrolase (converting enzyme).

    b. Activity
       1) <u>Angiotensin I</u>: rapidly converted to angiotensin II following an intravenous dose; less than 1% as potent as angiotensin II on smooth muscle, heart or adrenal cortex.
       2) <u>Angiotensin II</u>: most potent form
       3) <u>Angiotensin III</u>: 25% as potent as angiotensin II in elevating blood pressure; 10% as potent in stimulating the adrenal medulla; equipotent as angiotensin II in stimulating aldosterone secretion.
    c. Functions
       1) <u>Cardiovascular System</u>: vasoconstriction and increased blood pressure; increased force of cardiac contraction
       2) <u>Adrenal Cortex</u>: stimulates the synthesis and secretion of aldosterone
       3) <u>Kidney</u>: normally produces antidiuresis and antinatriuresis by: 1) constricting the arterioles surrounding the glomerulus, 2) decreasing the permeability of the filtration apparatus, and 3) stimulating Na^+/H^+ exchange in the proximal tubule
       4) <u>Autonomic Nervous System</u>: facilitates sympathetic transmission
       5) <u>Adrenal Medulla</u>: stimulates release of catecholamines
       6) <u>CNS</u>: may function as a neurotransmitter or neuromodulator
2. CONVERTING ENZYME INHIBITORS
    a. Inhibit the conversion of angiotensin I to angiotensin II
    b. Side effects include: a rapid decrease in blood pressure following the first dose in patients with severe hypertension or congestive heart failure, skin rash, loss of sense of taste, and dry cough
    c. Specific Agents
       1) Captopril
       2) Enalapril -- prodrug; more potent and longer duration
       3) Lisinopril -- long duration of action
    d. Therapeutic Uses
       1) Hypertension
       2) Chronic congestive heart failure

E. PROSTAGLANDINS (and related agents)

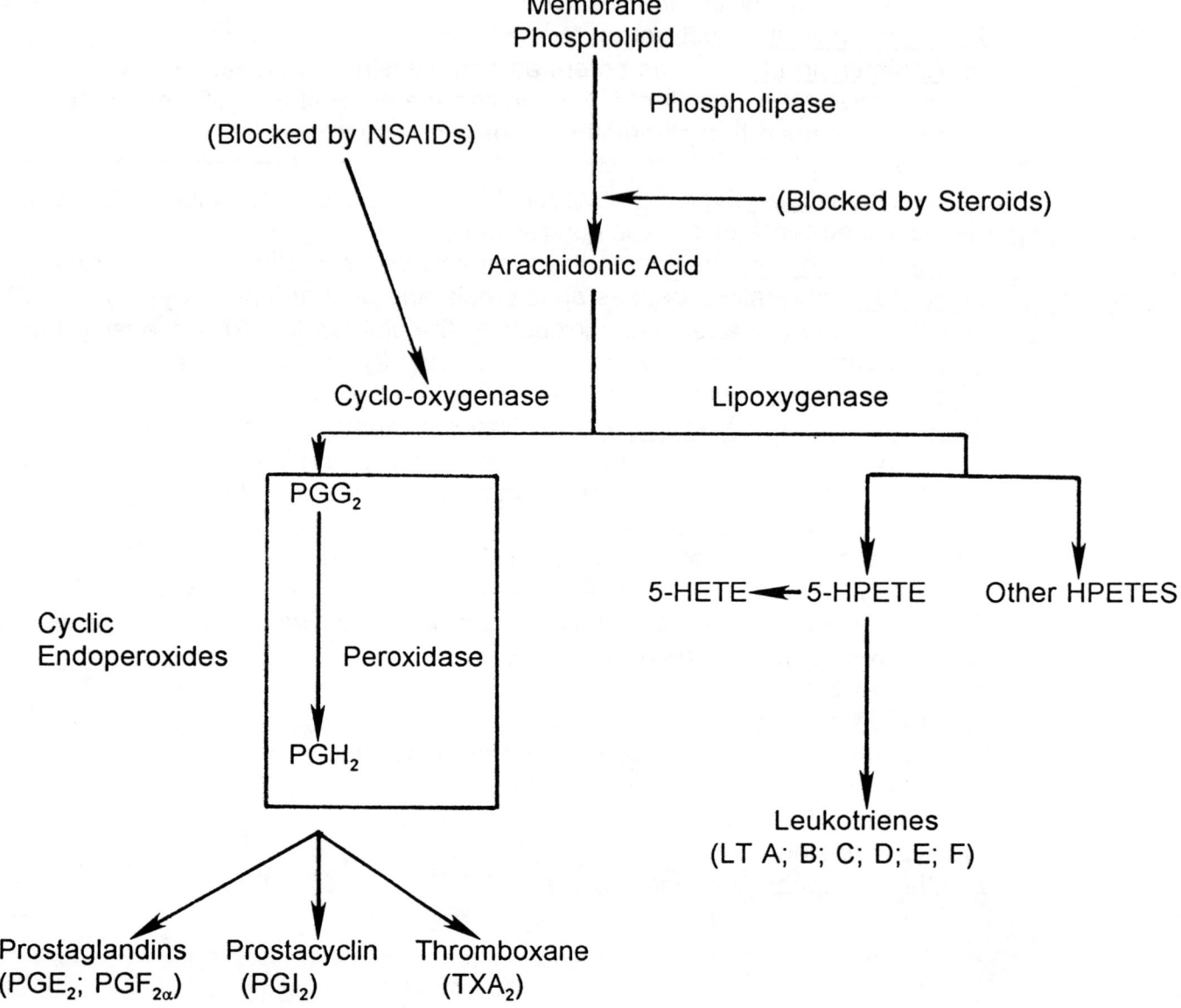

1. **GENERAL CONSIDERATIONS**
    a. Family of endogenous lipid substances; rapidly synthesized and degraded
    b. PGs have major effects on the: uterus, cardiovascular system, bronchi, GI tract, platelets, nervous system, and inflammatory and immune mechanisms
    c. NSAIDS block the synthesis of PGs by inhibiting cyclo-oxygenase and the formation of PGG_2 and PGH_2 which are precursors of all other PGs
    d. Lipoxygenase products are involved in cell mediated and immune mechanisms

2. IMPORTANT ACTIONS OF PGs, PROSTACYCLIN AND THROMBOXANES

System	PGEs	PGFs	Prostacyclin	Thromboxanes
Smooth muscle:				
Vascular	Dilation	Constriction	Dilation	Constriction
Bronchial	Dilation	Constriction		
Uterine	Contraction	Contraction		
GI	Contraction	Contraction		
Platelet aggregation	Inhibits ($\uparrow$ cAMP)		Inhibits ($\uparrow$ cAMP)	Stimulates ($\downarrow$ cAMP)
Gastric Acid Secretion	Decreases		Decreases	
Central NS	Fever Sedation			
Peripheral NS	Sensitizes nerve endings (pain)		Sensitizes afferent nerves (pain)	
Kidney	Renal blood flow Renin secretion Natriuresis			

3. THERAPEUTICS
   a. Abortificients (2nd trimester):
     1) PGE_2 (dinoprostone)
     2) $PGF_{2\alpha}$ (dinoprost tromethamine)
     3) 15-methyl $PGF_{2\alpha}$ (carboprost tromethamine)
   b. Anti-ulcer
     1) PGE_1 methyl ester (misoprostol)

II. NON-STEROIDAL ANTIINFLAMMATORY DRUGS (NSAIDs)

A. ANALGESIC, ANTIPYRETIC AND ANTIINFLAMMATORY AGENTS

1. INFLAMMATION
   a. Initial event for most painful conditions is a noxious stimulus that results in the destruction or injury of tissue
   b. Inflammation begins following sublethal injury to tissue; functions to remove noxious agents from the site of injury, to repair damage and to return tissue function to normal
   c. Clinical features of inflammation are: swelling, redness, heat, and pain
   d. Biochemical mediators of pain and inflammation include:
      1) Histamine: released from mast cells during antigen-antibody reactions; produces vasodilation and increased capillary permeability; sensitizes free nerve endings to painful stimuli
      2) Serotonin: increased permeability of the vasculature
      3) Prostaglandins: released in response to cell membrane disturbances; cyclo-oxygenase product of arachidonic acid metabolism; potent mediators of pain and inflammation
      4) Slow-Reacting Substance of Anaphylaxis (SRS-A): lipoxygenase product of arachidonic acid metabolism; changes vascular permeability
      5) Lysosomal Products: enzymatic and non-enzymatic factors that trigger mast cell degranulation
      6) Interleukin-1: produced by activated macrophages; involved in fever production
      7) Bradykinin: produces pain, vasodilation, edema

2. MECHANISM OF ACTION
   The analgesic, antiinflammatory and antipyretic properties of NSAIDs are attributed to their ability to inhibit prostaglandin synthesis by inhibiting the enzyme cyclo-oxygenase.

3. SPECIFIC AGENTS
   a. **Aspirin (Acetylsalicylic Acid, ASA)**
      1) Pharmacologic Effects
         a) Antipyretic Effects: result of peripherally mediated vasodilation and/or a centrally mediated resetting of the temperature control center in the hypothalamus
         b) Antiinflammatory and Analgesic Effects: maximal analgesia (650 mg); maximal antiinflammatory effects (up to 5 g)
         c) Cardiovascular System: no effects at therapeutic doses
         d) Respiratory System: no effects at therapeutic doses
         e) Gastrointestinal System: major side effects of salicylates (gastric distress, occult gastric bleeding, sudden acute hemorrhage)
         f) Blood: increased bleeding time due to inhibition of platelet aggregation
         g) Kidney: may cause the appearance of albumin casts, RBCs, and WBCs in the urine

129

h) <u>Liver</u>: dose-dependent alterations in liver function, changes usually are subclinical and reversible.
2) Absorption, Metabolism and Excretion
  a) Well absorbed following oral administration
  b) Rapidly metabolized by plasma esterases to salicylic acid and acetic acid
  c) Salicylate ion highly bound (80-90%) to plasma proteins
  d) Conjugation in the liver is primary route of metabolism
  e) Metabolites excreted in the urine
3) Contraindications
  a) <u>Ulcer</u>: gastric irritation may aggravate ulcers
  b) <u>Asthma</u>: possible aspirin intolerance
  c) <u>Diabetes</u>: high doses may lower plasma glucose
  d) <u>Gout</u>: low doses can exacerbate gouty arthritis; high doses have a uricosuric effect
  e) <u>Influenza</u>: increased risk of developing Reye's syndrome in children with influenza or chicken pox
4) Toxicity
  a) <u>Chronic Salicylism</u>: usually not life-threatening
  b) <u>Acute</u>: commonly occurs in children; is life-threatening; hyperventilation and respiratory alkalosis occur initially, followed by respiratory and metabolic acidosis; treatment is supportive

b. Acetaminophen
1) Pharmacologic Effects
  a) <u>Antipyretic Effects</u>: comparable to aspirin
  b) <u>Analgesic Effects</u>: comparable to aspirin; drug of choice for patients in whom aspirin is contraindicated
  c) <u>Antiinflammatory</u>: NO significant antiinflammatory properties; acetaminophen may have greater activity against CNS enzymes than enzymes in the periphery, accounting for its lack of antiinflammatory activity
  d) <u>Cardiovascular System</u>: no effects at therapeutic doses
  e) <u>Respiratory System</u>: no effects at therapeutic doses
2) Absorption, Metabolism and Elimination
  a) Well absorbed following oral administration
  b) Conjugation in the liver is primary route of metabolism
  c) Eliminated in urine by filtration and active proximal tubular secretion
3) Toxicity
  a) High therapeutic index; estimated that 6 g or more must be ingested for toxicity to occur
  b) <u>Hepatotoxicity</u> is most serious toxic effect; caused by accumulation of toxic metabolite
  c) Treat with <u>acetylcysteine or methionine</u> to inactivate toxic metabolite; only effective within 10-24 hrs of overdose

c. Phenylpropionic Derivatives (Ibuprofen, Naproxen, etc.)
1) Effective analgesic, antipyretic and antiinflammatory agents

    2) Fewer GI effects than aspirin

    3) More desirable pharmacokinetic properties than aspirin (i.e., longer half-lives and longer dosing intervals)

  d. Pyrazolone Derivatives (Phenylbutazone, Oxyphenbutazone)

    Use limited by serious side effects: blood dyscrasias and bone marrow suppression

  e. Acetic Acid Derivatives (Indomethacin, Sulindac, Tolmetin)

    Severe side effects have limited use of indomethacin: GI pain, severe headache and confusion (20-25%), aplastic anemia and thrombocytopenia

  f. Fenamates (Mefenamic Acid, Meclofenamate)

    Use limited by high incidence (25%) of GI symptoms

  g. Oxicams (Piroxicam)

    1) Advantage over other NSAIDs is pharmacokinetic; average half-life is 50 hrs; allows a single daily dose to be effective

    2) Side effects: inhibition of platelet aggregation, GI irritation, peripheral edema (rare), aplastic anemia (rare)

III. MISCELLANEOUS AGENTS FOR THE TREATMENT OF RHEUMATOID ARTHRITIS

A. GOLD SALTS (AURANOFIN)
1. Used to treat inflammatory conditions; NO analgesic or antipyretic effects
2. Only used when refractory to NSAIDs because of side effects: mucocutaneous lesions, blood dyscrasias, anaphylactoid reactions
3. May induce remission of rheumatoid arthritis; durations highly variable
4. Agents do inhibit prostaglandin synthesis; mechanism of inducing remission unknown

B. ANTIMALARIAL AGENTS (CHLOROQUINE, HYDROXYCHLOROQUINE)
1. Administered in combination with other antiinflammatory agents
2. Clinical improvement may require 3-6 months of therapy
3. Serious ocular toxicity associated with these agents

C. PENICILLAMINE (CUPRIMINE)
1. Immunosuppressive and immunostimulant properties
2. Only used when alternative treatments ineffective
3. Clinical improvement may require months of therapy
4. Skin rashes and GI symptoms are common side effects

IV. MISCELLANEOUS AGENTS FOR THE TREATMENT OF GOUT

A. URICOSURIC AGENTS (PROBENECID, SULFINPYRAZONE)
1. Block tubular reabsorption of uric acid
2. Indicated for chronic gout
3. Side effects: GI irritation, allergic reactions.

B. ALLOPURINOL
1. Inhibits xanthine oxidase to reduce the synthesis of uric acid
2. Indicated for chronic gout
3. Side effects: GI irritation, allergic reactions, blood dyscrasias

C. COLCHICINE
1. Inhibits mitotic activity, neutrophil migration and phagocytic activity in inflammed tissue
2. Indicated for <u>acute gouty arthritis</u>
3. Side effects: GI irritation, bone marrow depression, myopathy and alopecia with long term use

REVIEW QUESTIONS

ONE BEST ANSWER

1. The most serious toxic effect of acetaminophen overdose is:

   A. Nephrotoxicity
   B. CNS toxicity
   C. Cardiotoxicity
   D. Respiratory depression
   E. Hepatotoxicity

2. All of the following drugs are matched correctly with their corresponding side effects EXCEPT:

   A. Phenylbutazone -- blood dyscrasias
   B. Indomethacin -- severe headache and confusion
   C. Aspirin -- gastrointestinal irritation
   D. Acetaminophen -- respiratory depression
   E. Aspirin -- increased bleeding time

3. Therapeutic uses of H_1 antihistamines include treatment of:

   A. Allergic rhinitis
   B. Vertigo
   C. Motion Sickness
   D. Emesis
   E. All of the above

4. Which one of the following agents is an H_2 antihistamine?

   A. Terfenadine
   B. Diphenhydramine
   C. Ranitidine
   D. Chlorpheniramine
   E. Meclizine

5. Which one of the following agents is used as a prophylactic agent for the treatment of asthma?

   A. Diphenhydramine
   B. Cimetidine
   C. Famotidine
   D. Cromolyn Sodium
   E. Terfenadine

6. The **MOST** common side effect of H_1 antihistamines is:

   A. Skin rash
   B. Sedation
   C. Loss of sense of taste
   D. Hypotension
   E. Convulsions

7. All of the following are true of angiotensin II **EXCEPT**:

   A. Stimulates secretion of catecholamines
   B. Stimulates synthesis of aldosterone
   C. Increases peripheral vascular resistance
   D. Is activated by renin
   E. Facilitates sympathetic transmission

8. Which one of the following angiotensin converting enzyme inhibitors is a prodrug?

   A. Lisinopril
   B. Enalapril
   C. Misoprostol
   D. Captopril
   E. Ketanserin

9. All of the following agents may contribute to the carcinoid syndrome **EXCEPT**:

   A. Serotonin
   B. Renin
   C. Histamine
   D. Bradykinin
   E. Epinephrine

10. All of the following are true of bradykinin **EXCEPT**:

    A. Causes bronchodilation
    B. Is formed from a plasma $\alpha 2$ globulin precursor by kallikrein
    C. Causes pain upon subcutaneous injection
    D. Causes vasodilation
    E. May be involved in the local regulation of renal function

ONE BEST ANSWER

11. Which agent is used to treat <u>acute</u> gouty arthritis?

    A. Allopurinol
    B. Colchicine
    C. Probenecid
    D. Aspirin
    E. Sulfinpyrazone

12. Aspirin is contraindicated in the following patients:

    A. Asthmatics
    B. Children with influenza or chicken pox
    C. Ulcer patients
    D. Diabetics
    E. All of the above

13. The primary advantage of the oxicam class of NSAIDs is their:

    A. Increased oral bioavailability
    B. Long half-life
    C. Lower cost
    D. More effective analgesic properties

14. Gold salts used to treat rheumatoid arthritis:

    A. Are potent analgesics
    B. Have few side effects
    C. Are potent antipyretics
    D. May induce remission
    E. Are the drugs of choice for initial treatment of rheumatoid arthritis

15. Which one of the following agents inhibits xanthine oxidase to reduce the synthesis of uric acid?

    A. Probenecid
    B. Colchicine
    C. Allopurinol
    D. Indomethacin
    E. Sulfinpyrazone

16. All of the following signs and symptoms may be associated with acute salicylate toxicity **EXCEPT**:

    A. Hyperventilation
    B. Hypothermia
    C. Acid-base disturbances
    D. Gastrointestinal symptoms

17. All of the following drugs have significant anti-inflammatory properties **EXCEPT**:

    A. Acetaminophen
    B. Indomethacin
    C. Phenylbutazone
    D. Aspirin
    E. Piroxicam

18. The initial disturbance in acute aspirin toxicity is:

    A. Respiratory acidosis
    B. Respiratory alkalosis
    C. Metabolic acidosis
    D. Metabolic alkalosis
    E. Hypoventilation

19. Which one of the following prostaglandins or prostaglandin analogs is used clinically to inhibit gastric acid secretion?

    A. Dinoprostone
    B. Dinoprost tromethamine
    C. Carboprost
    D. Misoprostol
    E. Cytoprostol tromethamine

20. All of the following statements are true of PGEs **EXCEPT**:

    A. Dilation of bronchial smooth muscle
    B. Increased gastric acid secretion
    C. Inhibition of platelet aggregation
    D. Contraction of uterine smooth muscle
    E. Dilation of vascular smooth muscle

21. H_2 histamine receptors mediate:

    A. CNS stimulation
    B. Bronchoconstriction
    C. Gastric secretion
    D. Gastrointestinal tract contraction
    E. Pain and itching

22. Tissue release and production of histamine is stimulated by:

    A. Damage to cells and tissue
    B. Curare
    C. Morphine
    D. Snake venoms
    E. All of the above

ONE BEST ANSWER

23. The most effective treatment for anaphylactoid reactions is:

    A. Promethazine
    B. Epinephrine
    C. Terfenadine
    D. Ephedrine
    E. Histamine

24. Serotonin produces all of the following effects **EXCEPT**:

    A. Increased respiratory rate
    B. Decreased blood pressure
    C. Contraction of bronchial smooth muscle
    D. Increased motility of the small intestine
    E. Positive chronotropic effects on the heart

25. Which one of the following serotonin receptor antagonists is used therapeutically for the prophylactic treatment of migraines?

    A. Cyproheptadine
    B. Ketanserin
    C. Methysergide
    D. Chlorpromazine

26. Which one of the following H_2 histamine receptor antagonists inhibits cytochrome P450 and may potentiate other drugs?

    A. Famotidine
    B. Cimetidine
    C. Ranitidine
    D. Cromolyn sodium

27. Inhibition of cyclo-oxygenase might be expected to:

    A. Increase leukotriene levels
    B. Inhibit arachidonic acid levels
    C. Inhibit prostacyclin synthesis
    D. Increase cyclic endoperoxide levels

28. All of the following statements are true regarding prostacyclin **EXCEPT**:

    A. Dilation of vascular smooth muscle
    B. Increased gastric acid secretion
    C. Inhibition of platelet aggregation
    D. Sensitization of afferent nerves

29. All of the following produce therapeutic effects by interfering with prostaglandin synthesis **EXCEPT**:

    A. Acetaminophen
    B. Indomethacin
    C. Phenylbutazone
    D. Sulfinpyrazone
    E. Piroxicam

30. Betazole is a(n):

    A. H_1 agonist
    B. 5-HT_2 agonist
    C. H_2 agonist
    D. B_2 agonist

31. Which one of the following antihistamines has been reported to interact with inhibitors of drug metabolism to promote arrhythmias?

    A. Loratidine
    B. Terfenadine
    C. Tripelennamine
    D. Clemastine

MATCHING: Questions 32-42.

Match the drugs with their principal use:

A. Meclizine
B. Dinoprostone
C. Cimetidine
D. Renin
E. Colchicine
F. Diphenhydramine
G. Acetaminophen
H. Terfenadine
I. Cyproheptadine
J. Promethazine

K. Angiotensin II
L. Acetylcysteine
M. Captopril
N. Ketanserin
O. Nedocromil sodium
P. Aspirin
Q. Methysergide
R. Penicillamine
S. Allopurinol
T. Probenecid

32. Prevention of motion sickness

33. Treatment of allergic symptoms when drowsiness must be avoided

34. Prophylactic treatment of asthma

35. Treatment of duodenal ulcers

36. Treatment of carcinoid syndrome

37. Prophylactic treatment of migraine headaches

38. Treatment of acute gouty arthritis

39. Treatment of fever in a child with chicken pox

40. Treatment of renin-produced hypertension

41. 2nd trimester abortifacient

42. Treatment of acetaminophen overdose

CHAPTER 8: <u>THE ENDOCRINE SYSTEM</u>

I. THYROID - ANTITHYROID

A. TREATMENT OF HYPOTHYROIDISM

1. Natural hormones are thyroxine (T_4) and triiodothyronine (T_3). T_4 has a slower onset, is more extensively bound to plasma proteins and has a longer duration than T_3. T_3 is four times more potent than T_4.

2. Synthetic hormones (LEVOTHYROXINE and LIOTHYRONINE) or glandular extracts (THYROID) are used for replacement therapy. Levothyroxine is the drug of choice.

3. Uses
   a. Hypothyroidism, regardless of etiology: congenital (cretinism), autoimmune thyroiditis (e.g., Hashimoto's), during pregnancy and postpartum.
   b. Thyroid carcinoma (to suppress TSH).

4. Overdosage causes tachycardia, palpitations, restlessness, tremor, cardiac arrhythmias.

B. TREATMENT OF HYPERTHYROIDISM

1. Inhibitors of Hormone Synthesis
   a. PROPYLTHIOURACIL and METHIMAZOLE act by inhibiting the iodination of tyrosyl residues in thyroglobulin and the coupling of iodotyrosines. Methimazole is more potent and has a longer duration than propylthiouracil. Effects are not apparent until thyroid reserve is depleted.
   b. These drugs cross the placenta and are excreted into milk (propylthiouracil less than methimazole); babies should have thyroid function monitored.
   c. Remission may be produced, but relapse occurs frequently.
   d. Agranulocytosis is the most serious untoward reaction; rash is the most common.

2. Iodine (LUGOL'S SOLUTION, POTASSIUM IODIDE)
   a. Iodine (supraphysiological dose) produces temporary remission; used in thyrotoxic crisis, before surgery (to decrease vascularity of gland) or after radioiodine.
   b. Its main effect is to inhibit hormone release; effect is not sustained.

3. Radioiodine (SODIUM IODIDE-I^{131})
   a. Radioiodine accumulates in thyroid gland and destroys parenchymal cells; clinical improvement may take 2 to 3 months.

b. It is the preferred treatment for most patients with hyperthyroidism.
c. Subsequent hypothyroidism occurs in 20 to 80%.

    4. Adrenergic Blocking Agents (e.g., propranolol, atenolol, esmolol, metoprolol)
       a. They control symptoms; are used to treat/prevent thyrotoxicosis; not used alone.

II. ADRENOCORTICAL STEROIDS

A. GLUCOCORTICOIDS

1. The natural glucocorticoid cortisol has some salt retaining activity.

2. Synthetic hormones are effective orally, parenterally, topically.
   a. Short-acting
     HYDROCORTISONE (cortisol)
   b. Intermediate-acting
     PREDNISONE
     METHYLPREDNISOLONE
     TRIAMCINOLONE
   c. Long-acting
     DEXAMETHASONE
     BETAMETHASONE
   d. For local use
     BECLOMETHASONE
     FLUOCINONIDE

3. Effects
   a. Metabolic: glucocorticoids stimulate hepatic gluconeogenesis, diminish peripheral glucose utilization, promote glycogen synthesis, increase proteolysis and release amino acids for gluconeogenesis; they cause hyperglycemia, fatty acid mobilization, fat redistribution and protein catabolism.
   b. Anti-inflammatory: glucocorticoids inhibit every step of inflammatory process, including neutrophil actions, eicosanoid release and late-phase allergic reactions.
   c. Immunosuppressive

4. Uses
   a. Replacement therapy: glucocorticoids (usually hydrocortisone) are used to treat adrenocortical insufficiency; a salt-retaining hormone may also be needed.
   b. Congenital adrenal hyperplasia: glucocorticoids are used to suppress ACTH.

c. Therapy of non-endocrine diseases:

1) Rheumatoid arthritis
2) Leukemia, lymphoma
3) Allergic reactions
4) Asthma
5) Inflammatory and autoimmune disorders
6) Immunosuppression for transplantation
7) Collagen disorders
8) Cerebral edema
9) Bacterial meningitis

5. Adverse effects

Large doses of glucocorticoids for 1 week or less do not pose problems, but patients with nonendocrine disorders who receive systemic corticosteroids for longer times develop adverse effects, including suppression of the HPA axis and:

a. Hyperglycemia
b. Increased susceptibility to infection
c. Weight gain, Cushingoid features
d. Osteoporosis
e. Behavioral/personality changes
f. Myopathy
g. Ocular effects
h. Growth retardation in children

When possible, glucocorticoids should be administered locally to minimize adverse effects, or alternate-day therapy should be used.

B. MINERALOCORTICOIDS

1. The major mineralocorticoid produced by the adrenal gland is aldosterone; it has a very short half-life and is not used therapeutically.

2. FLUDROCORTISONE, a synthetic steroid, is the only orally-effective mineralocorticoid; it is used in salt-losing forms of adrenal insufficiency.

3. Mineralocorticoids promote sodium reabsorption by the distal tubules; potassium and hydrogen ions are excreted in exchange. They help maintain normal blood volume.

C. TREATMENT OF ADRENOCORTICAL HORMONE HYPERSECRETION

1. Inhibitors of adrenocortical hormone synthesis are used to treat Cushing's syndrome, adrenal adenoma or carcinoma, and ectopic ACTH-producing tumors.

   a. KETOCONAZOLE inhibits several adrenal hydroxylases (P450's), is the agent of choice for blocking cortisol synthesis.
   b. AMINOGLUTETHIMIDE blocks the conversion of cholesterol to pregnenolone, decreases secretion of all adrenal steroids.
   c. METYRAPONE blocks cortisol synthesis by inhibiting 11β-hydroxylase.
   d. MITOTANE specifically destroys adrenal cortical cells, which decreases the synthesis of adrenal steroids.

2. SPIRONOLACTONE is an receptor antagonist; it competes with aldosterone, is used to treat primary hyperaldosteronism.

III. PARATHYROID HORMONE AND OTHER FACTORS AFFECTING BONE METABOLISM

A. PTH MAINTAINS BLOOD CALCIUM BY:

1. Affecting mobilization of bone calcium
2. Affecting absorption of calcium by gut
3. Affecting excretion of calcium by kidney
4. Increasing formation of active vitamin D3 ($1,25(OH)_2D$) by kidney

B. PTH not used often therapeutically because same effect obtained with doses of vitamin D or its derivatives.

C. Vitamin D derivatives have well established actions on absorption of calcium from gut and reabsorption of bone.

D. OTHER HORMONAL REGULATORS

1. Calcitonin acts on bone and kidney to decrease calcium in blood; used in Paget's disease, hypercalcemia and osteoporosis
2. Glucocorticoids: enhance bone loss
3. Estrogens: prevent accelerated bone loss postmenopausally but do not restore bone

E. NONHORMONAL AGENTS

1. Etidronate - diphosphonate which inhibits bone resorption
2. Fluorides - treat osteoporosis
3. Plicamycin (mithramycin) - inhibits osteoclast function in treatment of hypercalcemia, highly toxic

IV. INSULIN

A. Used in treatment of insulin-dependent diabetic patients (IDDM) and some individuals with noninsulin-dependent diabetes (NIDDM).

B. Preparations made from beef or pork pancreas; or human insulin made either semisynthetically from pork insulin or completely synthetically by recombinant DNA techniques. Human insulin absorbed more quickly than pork insulin. Insulin has a short half-life and preparations have been developed to delay absorption and prolong its action. The unmodified, rapidly acting insulin is regular insulin. The modified preparations are:

1. Addition of protamine to form a slowly absorbed complex; NPH (isophane) insulin-termed intermediate in rate of onset and duration of action. No long acting preparation approved
2. Different sizes of crystals-lente series; semilente (short), lente (intermediate) and ultralente (long)

C. Insulin controls hyperglycemia and ketoacid formation by several mechanisms including:

   1. Increased transport of glucose into fat and muscle, increased muscle and hepatic glycogen synthesis
   2. Inhibition of lipolysis, increased triglyceride synthesis
   3. Inhibition of protein catabolism; increased amino acid transport and ribosomal protein synthesis
   4. Decreased hepatic glucose production (gluconeogenesis)
   5. Decreased glucagon secretion

D. Insulin therapy may have no effect on cardiovascular lesion associated with chronic insulin deficiency

E. Untoward reactions:

   1. Onset of hypoglycemia in well-controlled patients
      a. Causes
         1) wrong dose
         2) exercise inappropriate for dose of insulin; exercise increases glucose uptake by insulin-independent mechanisms
         3) not eating at regular time or eating insufficient amounts
         4) drugs enhancing insulin-induced hypoglycemia include: anabolic steroids, captopril, ethyl alcohol and salicylates
      b. Treatment
         1) treat with i.v. glucose if available
         2) patients may be instructed in the use of glucagon for treating reactions
         3) beta-adrenergic blocking drugs may mask symptoms of hypoglycemia and delay onset of treatment; these drugs also impair counter-regulatory responses
   2. Allergic reactions and localized atrophy less common with newer single component insulin preparations

F. Insulin antagonists:

   1. Glucocorticoids
   2. Pregnancy and birth control pills
   3. Weight gain
   4. Infections
   5. Surgical procedures
   6. Some drugs including thiazide diuretic agents and calcium channel blockers

G. Treatment of ketoacidosis includes:

   1. I.V. insulin
   2. Hypotonic saline - need to replenish and maintain intravascular volume
   3. Sometimes bicarbonate - only if pH is below 7.0
   4. Sometimes KCl - more often than not; whole body potassium low even with normokalemia
   5. Sometimes phosphate - only if hypophosphatemic
   6. Get glucose below 250 mg%, but not too rapidly in order to avoid cerebral edema

H. Oral hypoglycemic agents:

   1. Used in the treatment of NIDDM although diet and exercise are the primary treatments of this syndrome. One study (UGDP) found an increased incidence of cardiovascular deaths with use of these drugs, but the design and conclusions are in dispute and not confirmed in other studies.
   2. Sulfonylurea derivatives (tolbutamide, chlorpropamide, glipizide, glyburide and others)
      a. Mechanism of action
         1) Release insulin from pancreas. Primary mechanism considered to be closure of specific channels for potassium ion. Depolarization results and calcium ions enter. Amount of insulin release modified by concurrent changes in cyclic-AMP and protein kinase C.
         2) Might also have effects on liver as gluconeogenesis is decreased.
         3) Increase number of insulin receptors on cells
         4) Decrease circulating glucagon
      b. Differences in duration between derivatives depend on rate of metabolism by the liver and type of metabolites; i.e., active or inactive; Chlorpropamide metabolized slowest (t½ 36 hr)
      c. Can interact with other drugs by:
         1) Protein binding displacement; less a factor with second generation agents
         2) Changes in microsomal drug metabolism
         3) Decreased renal excretion of active metabolites

4) Additive effects on glucose disposition (i.e., aspirin)
5) Ethanol may increase or decrease hypoglycemic action; disulfiram-like effect possible
d. Useful only in non-insulin requiring diabetics, failure of therapy with continued use occurs (secondary failure)
e. Adverse reactions
1) Hypoglycemia
2) Granulocytopenia
3) Cholestatic jaundice
4) Allergic reactions
5) Chlorpropamide may cause water retention because of augmentation of ADH action

3. Biguanide derivatives (phenformin and metformin)
a. Phenformin was removed from use by the FDA because of a high incidence of lactic acidosis. Phenformin has been available by special dispensation from the FDA. Metformin has been used in Europe for 30 years and should be on the U.S. market by 1995.
b. Mechanism of action
1) do NOT increase release of pancreatic insulin, therefore the risk of hypoglycemia is less than that found for the sulfonylurea agents. These compounds also are ineffective in IDDM.
2) decrease hepatic gluconeogenesis and absorption of glucose from the G.I. tract.
3) unlike the sulfonylurea agents, metformin does not cause weight gain probably because the insulin concentration is lower.
c. Adverse reactions
1) G.I. disturbances including diarrhea
2) Smaller risk of lactic acidosis with metformin than that found with phenformin; however, metformin is contraindicated in patients with heart, liver or renal disease.

V. OVARIAN HORMONES AND OVULATORY AGENTS

A. ESTROGENS

1. Several types of estrogen preparations are available. Effectiveness by oral route depends on extent of metabolism by liver.
a. ESTRADIOL (estradiol esters for i.m. injection, transdermal patch)
b. CONJUGATED ESTROGENS (oral, parenteral, topical); Premarin® contains estrone and equilin
c. Synthetic steroids (oral): ETHINYL ESTRADIOL, MESTRANOL
d. Nonsteroidal synthetics (oral, parenteral): DIETHYLSTILBESTROL

2. Estradiol is the major estrogen in premenopausal women. Together with progesterone, estrogen maintains reproductive tissues and processes. Estrogen also has important effects on metabolism, e.g., transport proteins, clotting factors, electrolyte balance, serum lipids.

3. Unless the uterus has been removed, estrogens are usually administered in cyclic fashion with a progestin. Estrogen is used:
    a. For contraception - it's major use.
    b. To supplement inadequate production, e.g., constitutional delay of puberty, ovariectomy, menopause, osteoporosis.
    c. To correct hormonal imbalance, e.g., dysfunctional uterine bleeding.
    d. To reverse an abnormal process, e.g., hirsutism, endometriosis.

4. Adverse effects
    a. Nausea and vomiting, breast tenderness, and weight gain due to sodium and water retention - usually disappear with continued administration.
    b. Increased risk of endometrial cancer - is prevented by addition of a progestin.
    c. Reproductive tissue abnormalities and cancers in DES daughters and sons
    d. Gallstones
    e. Replacement dosages do not produce adverse cardiovascular effects.

B. PROGESTINS

1. Preparations
    a. PROGESTERONE, the natural hormone, is available in an oily solution for injection.
    b. Most preparations are synthetic steroids, e.g., NORETHINDRONE, ETHYNODIOL, NORGESTREL (oral) and MEDROXYPROGESTERONE (oral, parenteral). Some have sight androgenic activity.

2. With estrogen, progesterone supports female reproductive tissues and processes, and is especially important for maintaining pregnancy. Progesterone withdrawal is the primary signal for the onset of menstruation.

3. Uses
    a. Contraception - major use
    b. Dysfunctional uterine bleeding
    c. Dysmenorrhea, endometriosis - with estrogen, to suppress ovulation

4. Adverse reactions
    Decreased HDL - androgenic preparations

C. ANTIPROGESTINS

MIFEPRISTONE (RU-486) is a potent competitive antagonist of progesterone.

When administered in the follicular phase of the menstrual cycle, the drug prevents ovulation by inhibiting the effects of progesterone on the pituitary or hypothalamus. When given later, the drug terminates pregnancy by blocking the actions of progesterone on the uterus. Mifepristone is also a glucocorticoid antagonist.

D. HORMONAL CONTRACEPTION

1. Combination oral contraceptives
   a. Combination OC's contain a synthetic estrogen and a progestin; monophasic, biphasic and triphasic preparations are available.
   b. They act by inhibiting ovulation through negative feedback effects and by thickening the cervical mucus.
   c. Most adverse effects are related to the estrogen component (see above), but cardiovascular changes may be caused by either component.
   d. Adverse reactions other than those associated with estrogen therapy include:
      1) breakthrough bleeding with low estrogen preparations
      2) abnormal glucose tolerance
      3) alterations in serum lipids
      4) thromboembolic disease (minimal in low estrogen preparations)
      5) hypertension

2. Progestin only contraceptives
   a. Progestin only "minipills" contain lower doses of progestin than combination OC's and are taken daily. Subdermal implants steadily release small doses of progestin.
   b. These preparations do not inhibit ovulation consistently; their contraceptive actions are due to formation of an impenetrable cervical mucus and to endometrial involution.
   c. Unpredictable bleeding is a common side effect.

E. OVULATORY AGENTS

1. CLOMIPHENE
   a. Clomiphene is an antiestrogen with weak estrogenic activity.
   b. It acts by binding estrogen receptors and preventing the normal feedback inhibition by estrogen of GnRH and gonadotropin secretion. Ovarian stimulation and ovulation result.
   c. Adverse reactions
      1) mild menopausal symptoms
      2) ovarian cyst formation
      3) multiple births

2. MENOTROPINS (human menopausal gonadotropins)
   a. Menotropins, made from urine of post-menopausal women, contains both FSH and LH; hCG is added to induce ovulation. Menotropins is also used to treat male infertility.
   b. Adverse reactions
      1) multiple births
      2) ovarian enlargement with possible pain and ascites

3. BROMOCRIPTINE inhibits prolactin secretion, corrects infertility (male and female) secondary to hyperprolactinemic states.

4. GONADORELIN, a synthetic GnRH, may be used in lieu of menotropins. It is administered in pulsatile fashion using a portable pump.

VI. ANDROGENS AND ANABOLIC STEROIDS

A. ANDROGENIC/ANABOLIC AGENTS

1. Preparations
   a. Unaltered testosterone is not suitable for oral or parenteral administration because of rapid absorption and hepatic metabolism.
   b. TESTOSTERONE esters, e.g., testosterone cypionate, testosterone enanthate, dissolved in oily solutions and given i.m., are preferred for replacement therapy.
   c. Synthetic androgens, e.g., FLUOXYMESTERONE, METHYLTESTOSTERONE, and DANAZOL, contain 17α-alkyl substitutions to retard hepatic degradation and are orally effective. The substituted androgens produce liver dysfunction.
   d. Anabolic steroids, e.g., OXYMETHALONE, OXANDROLONE, also contain 17α-alkyl substitutions. They are weak androgens designed to provide anabolic activity; it is impossible to completely separate androgenic and anabolic effects.

2. Uses
   a. Hypogonadism (primary, secondary or tertiary) - testosterone esters
   b. Constitutional delay of growth - androgenic or anabolic steroids
   c. Endometriosis - danazol
   d. Hereditary angioneurotic edema - 17α-alkylated compounds

3. Adverse Effects
   a. Androgenic effects: acne, facial hair, deepening of voice are earliest; priapism; prostatic hyperplasia
   b. Gynecomastia
   c. Cholestatic hepatitis - 17α-alkylated compounds
   d. Atherogenic changes in blood lipids - with large doses taken by athletes
   e. Sodium retention and edema
   f. Benign and malignant tumors of the liver (rare)

B. ANTIANDROGENS

Antiandrogens may be useful for the treatment of hirsutism, precocious puberty, prostatic hyperplasia, prostate cancer, sex offenders.

1. CYPROTERONE has both antiandrogenic and progestational activity.
2. FLUTAMIDE is a competitive antagonist of testosterone.
3. FINASTERIDE blocks the conversion of testosterone to dihydrotestosterone by inhibiting the enzyme 5-α reductase.

VII. ANTERIOR PITUITARY AND HYPOTHALAMUS

A. GROWTH HORMONE

1. Hypothalamus
   a. Growth hormone-releasing factor (GHRH): a truncated protein (GHRH$_{44}$) is available for investigational use in the diagnosis and treatment of growth hormone deficiency.
   b. Growth hormone release-inhibiting hormone (somatostatin): an 8-amino acid analog (octreotide) approved for clinical use.
      1) inhibits not only the secretion of growth hormone but also TSH, insulin, glucagon and vasoactive intestinal peptide (VIP)
      2) approved for treatment of carcinoid tumors and vipoma
      3) improves clinical symptoms in acromegaly, insulinoma and glucagonoma
      4) low incidence of GI toxicity
2. Anterior Pituitary-Somatrem and somatropin: purified polypeptide of recombinant DNA origin used to treat growth hormone deficiency

B. ADRENOCORTICOTROPIN

1. Hypothalamus - Corticotropin - releasing hormone: investigational for differential diagnosis of site of hormone production in Cushing's disease
2. Anterior pituitary - ACTH
   a. Too short acting for most treatments
   b. Test for adrenal insufficiency
   c. Test for adrenal carcinoma

C. FSH AND LH - USE HCG AND HMG (See Ovulatory Agents)

D. GONADOTROPIN RELEASING HORMONE (GNRH) - (synthetic analogs)

1. Leuprolide (LHRH)- chronic treatment decreases LH and FSH secretion
   a. Given i.m. to treat endometriosis
   b. Used to treat prostatic carcinoma
2. Narfarelin
   a. Used intranasally for endometriosis
   b. May cause bone loss through a prolonged hypoestrogenic state
   c. This drug and leuprolide may be better than danazol for the treatment of endometriosis because they lack androgenic action

E. THYROID - STIMULATING HORMONE

1. Hypothalamus - thyrotropin-releasing hormone (TRH; protirelin): used to diagnose hyper- and hypothyroid states
2. Anterior pituitary - thyrotropin (TSH): diagnostic use largely replaced by TRH; used to stimulate ^{131}I uptake in treatment of metastatic thyroid carcinoma

F. PROLACTIN

1. Hypothalamus - Loss of prolactin-inhibiting hormone (dopamine) after hypothalamic destruction associated with hypersecretion (amenorrhea/galactorrhea).
2. Anterior pituitary - no prolactin analogs; inhibition of secretion by bromocriptine
   a. Bromocriptine
      1) dopamine analog
      2) uses
         a) prolactin-secreting adenomas
         b) amenorrhea/galactorrhea
         c) suppress physiologic lactation
         d) acromegaly-adjunct to surgery or irradiation, causes a partial suppression of growth hormone secretion to await outcome of other treatments.
         e) other
            (1) Parkinson's disease
            (2) Cocaine withdrawal

VIII. POSTERIOR PITUITARY HORMONES

A. VASOPRESSIN (Antidiuretic Hormone) (See Section V for vasopressin discussion)

B. OXYTOCIN (See Section VIII for other oxytocic drugs)

1. Both hormones are synthesized in the hypothalamus, and are transported to the posterior pituitary where they are stored.
2. Both are peptide hormones consisting of 9 amino acids, and they differ only in the amino acids at positions 3 and 8.
3. Both have a short half-life (15-30 min).
4. Because of their chemical similarities, vasopressin has slight oxytocic activity, and oxytocin has slight antidiuretic activity. However, oxytocin has no vasoconstricting activity.
5. Posterior pituitary injection contains both hormones, but is seldom used because pure vasopressin and oxytocin are available.

REVIEW QUESTIONS

ONE BEST ANSWER

1. Propylthiouracil decreases the secretion of thyroxine by:

   A. Inhibiting the uptake of iodide by the thyroid gland
   B. Interfering with the secretion of TSH by the pituitary
   C. Interfering with the synthesis of thyroid hormone
   D. Inhibiting the synthesis of thyroglobulin
   E. Inhibiting the deiodination of T4

2. All of the following are true statements concerning the use of large doses of Vitamin D in the treatment of hypoparathyroidism EXCEPT:

   A. It increases the mobilization of calcium from bone
   B. It decreases the excretion of calcium by the kidney
   C. It enhances the absorption of calcium from the gastrointestinal tract
   D. It increases the secretion of calcitonin

3. Clomiphene has been used in women for the treatment of infertility because it:

   A. Increases the secretion of FSH and LH
   B. Resembles diethylstilbestrol structurally
   C. Increases the chance that a fertilized ovum will be implanted
   D. Increases libido in ovulating women
   E. Inhibits androgen production by the adrenals

4. Which one of the following inhibitors does NOT act by inhibiting the synthesis of adrenocortical steroids?

   A. Aminoglutethimide
   B. Ketoconazole
   C. Metyrapone
   D. Spironolactone
   E. Mitotane

5. Severe adverse reactions are a therapeutic problem in the use of adrenal glucocorticoids in all of the following conditions EXCEPT:

   A. Suppression of the inflammatory reaction in collagen diseases
   B Treatment of acute and chronic lymphocytic leukemias
   C. Acute treatment of anaphylactic shock
   D. Treatment of severe chronic bronchial asthma
   E. Treatment of rheumatoid arthritis

6. Dexamethasone produces which one of the following metabolic changes?

   A. Decrease in hepatic glycogen storage
   B. Hypoglycemia
   C. Decrease in protein breakdown
   D. Increase in gluconeogenesis
   E. Increase in peripheral utilization of glucose

7. Which one of the following is associated with severe insulin deficiency?

   A. High plasma sodium ion concentrations
   B. Increased triglyceride synthesis
   C. Increased release of oxygen from red blood cells
   D. Decreased beta-hydroxybutyrate/acetoacetate ratio in plasma
   E. Sustained loss of skeletal muscle protein

8. Which of the following has been associated with the use of orally-effective androgenic steroids?

   A. Increase in nitrogen retention and muscle mass
   B. Stimulation of growth of a latent prostatic carcinoma
   C. Increased sodium retention and formation of edema fluid
   D. Cholestatic jaundice (17-alkyl derivatives)
   E. All of the above

ONE BEST ANSWER

9. A difference between methimazole and propylthiouracil is that:

A. Methimazole has a longer duration of action than propylthiouracil
B Methimazole inhibits thyroid hormone synthesis; propylthiouracil does not
C. Propylthiouracil crosses the placenta more readily than methimazole
D. Agranulocytosis is the most common adverse effect of propylthiouracil, whereas rash is the most common side effect of methimazole
E. Methimazole cannot be used with a beta-blocking agent.

10. Radioactive iodine in treatment of hyperthyroidism:

A. Causes a high incidence of hypothyroidism
B. Is rapidly and efficiently trapped by the thyroid
C. Is indicated in older patients with heart disease
D. Is contraindicated during pregnancy
E. All of the above

11. Levothyroxine toxicity is associated with:

A. Agranulocytosis
B. Increased plasma cholesterol concentrations
C. Depression
D. Cardiac symptoms
E. Aplastic anemia

12. Which one of the following is caused by methyltestosterone but not by testosterone propionate?

A. Facial hair
B. Acne
C. Deepening voice
D. Jaundice
E. Increased muscle strength

13. Prolonged administration of methylprednisolone may produce all of the following adverse effects EXCEPT:

A Behavioral and personality changes.
B. Cataracts
C. Osteoporosis
D. Myopathy
E. Hyponatremia and hyperkalemia

14. Which one of the following is the most life-threatening result of adrenal insufficiency?

A. Decreased gluconeogenesis
B Lymphoid hyperplasia
C. Inability to excrete a water load
D. Loss of sodium ion in the urine
E. Loss of potassium ion in the urine

15. Which one of the following drugs is the best choice for long-term treatment of hypogonadism in males?

A. Methyltestosterone
B. Testosterone cypionate
C. Fluoxymesterone
D. Danazol
E. Norethindrone

16. Estrogen therapy may be indicated for all of the following EXCEPT:

A. Failure of ovarian development
B. Carcinoma of the endometrium
C. Menopausal symptoms
D. Atrophic vaginitis
E. Prevention of osteoporosis

17. Which one of the following is an adverse effect of high dose estrogen therapy?

A. Acne
B. Lymphopenia
C. Weight loss
D. Thrombophlebitis

18. Which one of the following is responsible for the contraceptive action of the progestin-only minipill?

A. Inhibition of fertilization and implantation
B. Competitive inhibition of estradiol
C. Inhibition of ovulation
D. Enhancement of FSH and LH secretion

ONE BEST ANSWER

19. All of the following are true about therapeutic thyrotropin **EXCEPT**:

    A. Prepared from bovine anterior pituitaries
    B. Used in the diagnosis of hypothyroidism
    C. Used in therapy of metastatic thyroid carcinoma
    D. Can increase size and vascularity of thyroid gland
    E. Used with caution in presence of heart disease

20. The posterior pituitary hormones vasopressin and oxytocin share many similarities; in which of the following ways are they different?

    A. Site of biosynthesis
    B. Length of polypeptide chain
    C. Effect on uterine smooth muscle
    D. Effect of vascular smooth muscle
    E. Biological half-life

21. Oxytocin administration:

    A Induces vigorous contractions in the non-pregnant uterus which is in the secretory phase of the menstrual cycle
    B. Stimulates milk production in nursing mothers
    C. Is useful clinically for first trimester abortions
    D. Promotes diuresis
    E. Increases the frequency of contractions of the uterus late in pregnancy

22. All of the following are actions of insulin **EXCEPT**:

    A. Decreased mobilization of free fatty acids
    B. Increased uptake of glucose by muscle
    C. Increased rate of gluconeogenesis
    D. Increased formation of glycerophosphate by fat cells
    E. Increased hepatic glycogen synthesis

23. Which one of the following statements is true of the lente series of insulin preparations?

    A. These preparations are readily soluble and can be given I.V. to treat diabetic coma
    B. These preparations have effects qualitatively different from those of regular insulin
    C. This series of preparations includes long-acting human or beef insulin preparations
    D. These preparations are not associated with the development of antibodies to exogenously administered insulin
    E. Hyperglycemia occurs with overdose

24. Which one of the following is a true statement concerning the treatment of diabetic patients with metformin but **NOT** true of their treatment with sulfonylurea agents?

    A. Useful for the treatment of patients with IDDM
    B. Plasma insulin concentration does not increase during treatment
    C. Hepatic gluconeogenesis decreased
    D. Weight gain observed in many patients
    E. Ineffective in the absence of pancreatic insulin reserves

25. All of the following are actions of 1,25-dihydroxycholecalciferol **EXCEPT**:

    A. Is secreted by the kidneys
    B. Is derived from Vitamin D
    C. Stimulates intestinal calcium transport
    D. Stimulates calcium reabsorption from the bone matrix
    E. Toxicity is the result of hypocalcemia

26. All of the following could result in an alteration of the daily insulin dosage for a diabetic patient **EXCEPT**:

    A. Prolonged exercise
    B. Pregnancy
    C. Marked weight gain
    D. Glucocorticoid administration
    E. Treatment of hypertension with an α-adrenergic blocking drug

152

ONE BEST ANSWER

27. Therapy with a progestin may be indicated for which one of the following conditions?

    A. Dysfunctional uterine bleeding
    B. Hereditary angioneurotic edema
    C. Loss of appetite
    D. Elevated LDL cholesterol levels

28. Which one of the following is a mineralocorticoid?

    A. Fluocinonide
    B. Betamethasone
    C. Fludrocortisone
    D. Triamcinolone
    E. Prednisone

29. Adverse effects from glucocorticoid therapy may be minimized by:

    A. Use of smallest dose in emergency situation
    B. Alternate-day therapy
    C. Abrupt withdrawal after years of administration
    D. Use of largest dose for chronic disease

MATCHING: Use a letter only once:

    A. Estradiol
    B. Danazol
    C. Mestranol
    D. Norethindrone
    E. Progesterone

30. Weak androgen, used for endometriosis

31. Synthetic progestin, used alone in contraceptive "minipills"

32. Natural steroid that causes secretory endometrium; decline in activity is main signal for menstruation

33. Natural steroid that causes proliferative endometrium; decline in activity can bring about menstruation

34. Synthetic estrogen, used in combination oral contraceptives

MATCHING: Use a letter only once

    A. Lugol's solution
    B. Propylthiouracil
    C. Levothyroxine
    D. Liothyronine
    E. Propranolol

35. Therapeutic benefit is due to inhibition of thyroid hormone synthesis

36. Drug of choice for hypothyroidism

37. Therapeutic benefit is due to inhibition of thyroid hormone release and decrease in vascularity of the thyroid gland

38. Alleviates symptoms of hyperthyroidism without affecting the synthesis or secretion of thyroid hormones

MATCHING: Use a letter only once

    A. Hydrocortisone
    B. Metyrapone
    C. Prednisone
    D. Beclomethasone
    E. Spironolactone

39. Alternate day therapy for rheumatoid arthritis

40. Cushing's syndrome

41. Hyperaldosteronism

42. Aerosol therapy for bronchial asthma

43. Congenital adrenal hyperplasia

CHAPTER 9: ANTI-INFECTIVE AGENTS

I. INTRODUCTION TO CHEMOTHERAPY

Chemotherapeutic agents are intended to eliminate foreign organisms or abnormal cells from healthy tissues of the patient. An essential property of all chemotherapeutic drugs is selective toxicity; deleterious actions directed against the target cells without comparable effects on the tissue of the host. The degree of selective toxicity possessed by a drug is closely related to its mechanism of action. If a drug affects a vital process of parasitic cells, but which is not required in host tissue, the degree of selective toxicity can be quite good. The high incidence of adverse effects associated with most antiviral and antineoplastic drugs is directly related to the fact that these agents produce similar effects in both normal and target cells. Some examples of selective toxicity resulting from specific mechanisms of action are given in the following table:

Mechanism	"Selectively Toxic" Because:	Examples
Inhibition of cell wall synthesis	Mammalian cells have no cell walls	Penicillin Vancomycin
Inhibition of membrane function	Unique characteristics of fungal membranes	Nystatin Miconazole
Inhibition of protein synthesis	Specific binding sites on bacterial ribosome	Tetracycline Clindamycin
Inhibition of nucleic acid synthesis	Activity against unique enzymes (DNA gyrase; reverse transcriptase, etc.)	Ciprofloxacin Zidovudine Rifampin

Selective toxicity can also result when a drug is selectively transported into cells of the pathogen (tetracyclines and aminoglycosides, for example); or when the drug is activated by microbial enzymes to cytotoxic metabolites (nitrofurantoin).

Some chemotherapeutic drugs are classified as "antimetabolites"; substances which have structural similarity to substrates utilized in intermediary metabolism of the cell, and which compete for enzymatic binding sites. Examples are purine and pyrimidine analogs used in cancer or antiviral chemotherapy, or the sulfonamide antibacterial drugs. The ultimate effects of these "antimetabolites" may be exerted on nucleic acids, proteins, cell walls, etc.

Note that "selective toxicity" is not synonymous with drug safety. Most chemicals possess deleterious effects which are unrelated to their chemotherapeutic mechanism of action. Some of the agents cited in the table possess toxicities that limit their use to topical applications (nystatin), or to indications where less toxic agents are ineffective (vancomycin).

II. CHEMOTHERAPY OF MICROBIAL DISEASES

A. BETA-LACTAM ANTIBIOTICS

β-Lactam antibiotics have been widely investigated for use in medicine because of their high degree of selective toxicity against bacteria. Individual β-lactam antibiotics may differ widely in their antibacterial spectra, pharmacokinetic properties, and resistance to hydrolysis by β-lactamases.

Mechanism of action: All β-lactam antibiotics bind covalently to penicillin binding proteins (PBP's) of bacterial cell membranes. Various strains of bacteria may have differing numbers of PBPs, but all appear to be involved in some stage of bacterial cell wall synthesis. Incubation of susceptible bacteria with β-lactam antibiotics may result in morphological abnormalities and cell death. Cell lysis, when it occurs, may result from uncontrolled action of bacterial lytic enzymes. β-Lactam antibiotics may be bacteriostatic to some strains of bacteria at low drug concentrations. Because of the selective action of β-lactam antibiotics against cell wall synthesis, these drugs are most effective against actively growing bacterial cultures.

Metabolism and excretion: Most β-lactam antibiotics are excreted unchanged in the urine. Both glomerular filtration and tubular secretion contribute to the urinary secretion of β-lactam antibiotics; probenecid will inhibit tubular secretion. A few agents are excreted primarily into the bile.

Toxicity: Allergic reactions are the most common toxic complications, and there is a small incidence (5-10%) of cross-reactivity among the penicillins and cephalosporins. Some agents have unique toxicities of low incidence which are not characteristic of most β-lactam antibiotics. CNS dysfunction (lethargy, confusion, seizures) may occur with high blood and CSF levels.

Resistance: Many bacteria produce β-lactamase enzymes (e.g., penicillinase) which opens the β-lactam ring and destroys the activity of the antibiotic. Many cephalosporins are resistant to β-lactamases, and β-lactamase inhibitors combined with this class of antibiotics further extends their usefulness.

1. PENICILLINS:

a. <u>Narrow spectrum: Gram positive primarily are sensitive</u>
   1) PENICILLIN G (Benzyl penicillin) - The prototypic penicillin. It should be given parenterally because oral absorption is erratic due to instability in gastric acid. It can be combined with procaine or benzathine to prolong action after i.m. injection.
   2) PENICILLIN V (Phenoxymethyl penicillin) - Acid stable, for oral use only. Otherwise similar to penicillin G.
b. <u>Penicillinase-Resistant Penicillins</u> are also effective against gram-positive organisms, but remain useful if the bacteria produce penicillinase.
   Parenteral: METHICILLIN (prototype); oxacillin; nafcillin
   Oral: Oxacillin; cloxacillin; dicloxacillin; nafcillin
c. <u>"Extended Spectrum" Penicillins</u> possess activity against some important gram positive and gram-negative pathogens
   1) <u>Amino penicillins</u>: AMPICILLIN (prototype). AMOXICILLIN has superior absorption. Bacampicillin is hydrolyzed in the body to release ampicillin.
   2) "Anti-pseudomonal" penicillins: Ticarcillin and Carbenicillin.
d. <u>Broad Spectrum Penicillins</u> have improved activity against gram-negative pathogens, including <u>Pseudomonas aeruginosa</u>. Piperacillin, mezlocillin.

2. CEPHALOSPORINS: Includes the true cephalosporins (produced from <u>Cephalosporium</u> spp.) and cephamycins (produced from <u>Streptomyces</u> spp.). Cephamycins possess a 7-methoxy substitution on the β-lactam ring which results in greater resistance to β-lactamases. The possibility of chemical substitutions on both sides of the ring structure (R_1 and R_2) results in a number of agents with differing antibacterial spectra and pharmacokinetic properties. Loracarbef is a carbacephem, where the sulfur in the ring nucleus has been replaced with carbon. Cephalosporins are classified into "generations" on the basis of their microbial spectrum.

Cephalosporins

Cephamycins

a. <u>First-Generation Cephalosporins</u> - Most important for gram-positive activity. All are susceptible to β-lactamase inactivation.
   1) <u>Parenteral agents</u>: Cefazolin, Cephalothin, Cephapirin, Cephradine
   2) <u>Oral agents</u>: Cephalexin, Cefadroxil, Cephradine
   3) <u>Summary</u>: There are few important differences among the first generation cephalosporins. <u>CEFAZOLIN</u> has the longest half-life, reaches highest plasma levels after i.v. injection, and is least irritating of the parenteral agents, so is the best choice for i.m. injection. The absorption of <u>CEFADROXIL</u> after oral administration is somewhat greater than the other oral agents.
b. <u>Second-Generation Cephalosporins</u> - In general, have greater resistance to lactamases produced by gram-negative pathogens, especially <u>Hemophilus influenzae</u>, than first generation agents. However, first-generation agents are preferred for most gram-positive indications, and third-generation agents are usually more active against gram-negative pathogens.
   1) <u>Parenteral agents</u>: Cefamandole, Cefuroxime, Cefonicid, Cefoxitin, Cefotetan, Cefmetazole.
   2) <u>Oral agents</u>: Cefachlor, Cefuroxime axetil, Cefpodoxime proxetil, Cefprozil, Loracarbef.
   3) <u>Summary</u>: CEFOXITIN (a cephamycin) is probably the most notable drug of this class because of its good activity against anaerobic bacteria. Some individual features of other agents may make them useful in selected patients: long half-life (cefonicid); penetration into CSF (cefuroxime). Axetil and proxetil salts are hydrolyzed after absorption, and should be taken with food to achieve maximal blood levels.
c. <u>Third Generation Cephalosporins</u> - Broad spectrum antimicrobial drugs; however, potency against gram-positive microbes is generally inferior to first-generation agents. All third generation cephalosporins are resistant to hydrolysis by β-lactamases.

CEFOTAXIME	CEFTRIAXONE
CEFTAZIDIME	Cefoperazone
Cefixime	Ceftizoxime

Individual third generation cephalosporins have properties which may offer particular clinical advantages or unexpected toxicity. These properties are not necessarily shared by all third-generation cephalosporins. Cefixime is effective orally.
   1) <u>Advantageous properties</u>
      a) Penetration into CSF (Ceftazidime, Cefotaxime)
      b) Biliary excretion (Cefoperazone, Ceftriaxone)
      c) Long half-life (Ceftriaxone)
      d) Anti-pseudomonal activity (Ceftazidime)

2) Unusual toxicities
    a) Disulfiram-like effects (Cefoperazone)
    b) Hypoprothrombinemia (Possibly related to diminished synthesis of vitamin K by intestinal microbes, but is probably better explained by a chemical substituent on some cephalosporins (e.g., cefoperazone) which antagonizes prothrombin biosynthesis.)

3. CARBAPENEMS:

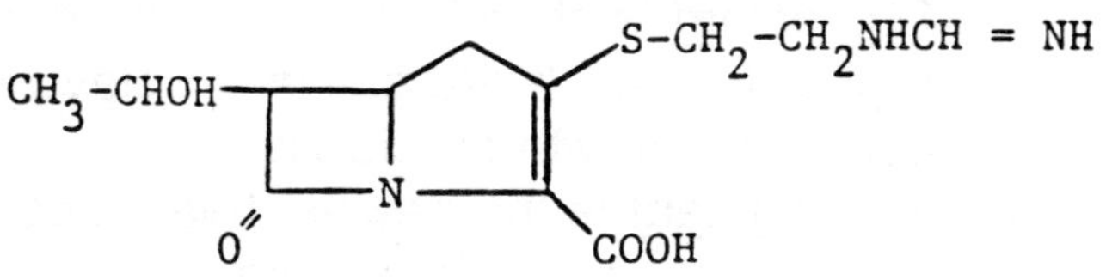

Imipenem

IMIPENEM was introduced in 1985 as the first "thienamycin" antibiotic to be marketed. Imipenem binds to all PBPs and has the broadest spectrum of any β-lactam antibiotic. It is also an irreversible β-lactamase inhibitor.

Imipenem is metabolized by a renal peptidase, and little active drug could be recovered in urine. To circumvent this metabolism, a specific inhibitor of the renal enzyme, cilistatin, was synthesized. Cilistatin also prevents renal toxicity sometimes observed with imipenem alone. A 1:1 combination of imipenem:cilistatin is the only form available.

Because of its broad spectrum, imipenem has many potential uses, but resistance can develop, especially among Pseudomonas species. Like other β-lactam antibiotics, imipenem has a low incidence of adverse reactions, but may trigger seizures in epileptic patients or in cases of head trauma.

4. MONOBACTAMS:

Monobactams are unusual β-lactam antibiotics in that the β-lactam ring is not fused with another ring. A number of monobactam antibiotics have been discovered, and are under study.

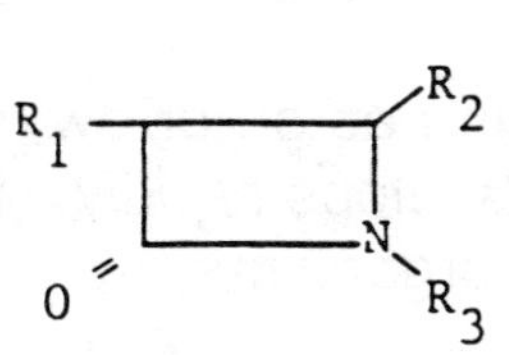

a. AZTREONAM: Aztreonam is a potent, narrow-spectrum antibiotic, with activity only against aerobic gram-negative bacteria. It is highly stable to β-lactamases, does not induce β-lactamase enzymes, and shows poor immune cross-reactivity with other β-lactam antibiotics. Aztreonam is synergistic with other β-lactam antibiotics and the aminoglycosides.

5. β-LACTAMASE INHIBITORS:

  a. <u>Clavulanic acid</u> is an oxapenem (in which the sulfur of the penicillin ring structure has been replaced with oxygen) which has poor antimicrobial activity, but is an irreversible inhibitor of many bacterial β-lactamases. Clavulanic acid is marketed in combination with other β-lactam antibiotics (amoxicillin, ticarcillin) to increase their effectiveness.
  b. <u>Sulbactam</u> is chemically derived from the penicillin ring structure. It has properties which are similar to clavulanic acid, and is marketed in combination with ampicillin.
  c. <u>Tazobactam</u> is the newest β-lactamase inhibitor, and is marketed in combination with piperacillin.

B. VANCOMYCIN

Vancomycin inhibits bacterial cell wall synthesis at a different step from β-lactam antibiotics, and is usually bactericidal. Bacteria seldom develop resistance to vancomycin. It should not be given i.m. because it causes tissue necrosis. When given i.v., it must be given slowly as a dilute solution to minimize thrombophlebitis, as well as flushing reactions associated with histamine release. Although it is not absorbed from the GI tract, vancomycin is indicated for susceptible pathogens in the bowel, such as treatment of antibiotic-associated pseudomembranous colitis.

C. MACROLIDE ANTIBIOTICS

Macrolide (large ring) antibiotics are characterized the presence of a 14- or 15-member lactone ring. Erythromycin is the prototype of these antibiotics, but newer macrolides possess improved pharmacokinetic properties and modest changes in the antibacterial spectrum.

<u>Mechanism of action:</u> Macrolides bind to the P site of the 50S bacterial ribosomal subunit. They block protein synthesis when a large amino acid or a polypeptide is in the P site.
<u>Spectrum:</u> Erythromycin has a narrow, gram-positive spectrum, similar to penicillin G. Resistance develops rapidly. Macrolides are also active against Chlamydia and Legionella organisms.

1. ERYTHROMYCIN:

Erythromycin is available as the base (unstable in acid), and as stearate, ethylsuccinate and estolate salts. The best absorption is obtained with the estolate salt. Erythromycin is distributed into total body water, but penetration into the CSF is poor, even when meninges are inflamed. The drug is extensively metabolized in the liver, so that dosage adjustments in renal failure are usually considered unnecessary.

Erythromycin is usually well tolerated, but many patients complain of gastric effects. Reversible intrahepatic obstructive jaundice may occur, especially with the estolate salt. Parenteral forms are highly irritating.

2. CLARITHROMYCIN:

Clarithromycin is a hydroxylated derivative of erythromycin, but is much better absorbed after oral administration. It is somewhat more active against gram-positive pathogens, Legionella, and Chlamydia than erythromycin.

3. AZITHROMYCIN:

Azithromycin has a 15-member lactone ring, and is more active than erythromycin against several gram-negative pathogens. The most unusual property of azithromycin is its uptake into a number of tissues (e.g., lung, tonsil, cervix), where it maintains high concentrations for prolonged periods. Azithromycin's long half-life allows once daily oral administration.

4. TROLEANDOMYCIN

Troleandomycin is seldom used because of its poor antibacterial properties and unfavorable pharmacokinetic properties.

D. LINCOMYCIN AND CLINDAMYCIN (7-chlorolincomycin)

1. Mechanism of action: The lincosamide antibiotics attach to 50S ribosomal subunit, at or near the erythromycin attachment site. They are chemically unlike, but pharmacologically similar to, erythromycin.
2. Antibacterial spectrum: Narrow gram-positive spectrum, but with excellent activity against anaerobic bacteria. Clindamycin is a more potent antimicrobial agent than lincomycin.
3. Absorption, distribution and excretion: Lincomycin is poorly absorbed after oral administration, and is seldom used clinically. The oral absorption of clindamycin is excellent, and is not affected by food. These drugs are widely distributed in the body (but reach only low concentrations in CSF, even when meninges are inflamed) and penetrate well into bone. Both drugs are metabolized extensively, and excreted primarily in bile and feces.
4. Toxicity: Diarrhea is most common adverse effect. Clindamycin is the antibiotic which has most frequently caused antibiotic-associated colitis. Skin rashes and reversible changes in hepatic enzymes in serum may also occur.
5. Uses: Clindamycin is useful for therapy of anaerobic infections, including those caused by Bacteroides fragilis. It is potentially useful as a penicillin substitute, but is more toxic than erythromycin.

E. CHLORAMPHENICOL

1. Mechanism of action: Chloramphenicol attaches at P sites of 50S subunit of microbial ribosomes and inhibits functional attachment of amino acyl end of AA-t-RNA to 50S subunit. The drug is bacteriostatic, not bactericidal.
2. Spectrum: Chloramphenicol is a broad spectrum antibiotic, more effective than tetracyclines against typhoid fever and other Salmonella infections. Good activity against many anaerobic bacteria and rickettsia.
3. Absorption, distribution, and excretion: Chloramphenicol is well absorbed after oral administration, and is distributed into total body water. Its high lipid solubility results in excellent penetration into CSF, ocular fluids and joint fluids. Chloramphenicol is rapidly excreted in urine, 10% as chloramphenicol, 90% as the glucuronide conjugate.
4. Toxicity: Irreversible aplastic anemia is a rare, but most serious effect. Reversible bone marrow depression may also occur. Gray baby syndrome in neonates is due to deficient glucuronidation of the drug and its subsequent accumulation in the infant's body. Superinfections by non-susceptible organisms are potential problems with all antibiotics, especially with broad-spectrum agents..
5. Uses: Chloramphenicol's broad spectrum and penetration into CSF make it useful in meningitis, rickettsial infections, anaerobic infections, and Salmonella infections. The risk of aplastic anemia limits its application to situations where safer drugs are not likely to be effective.

F. TETRACYCLINES

1. Mechanism of action: Tetracyclines preferentially bind to the 30S subunit of the microbial ribosome, and seem to interfere with binding of amino acyl-t-RNA and inhibit chain termination. Tetracyclines are usually bacteriostatic.
2. Spectrum: Tetracyclines are broad spectrum agents, effective against gram positive and gram negative bacteria, rickettsia, chlamydia, spirochetes, amebiasis.
3. Absorption, distribution, and excretion: Most tetracyclines are incompletely absorbed after oral administration, and absorption is further delayed by food, calcium salts, and aluminum salts. (Exception: The oral absorption of doxycycline is superior to the other tetracyclines, and is virtually unaffected by food.) Tetracyclines are distributed in total body water.

    Tetracyclines are usually excreted in the urine, so that renal function should be considered for dosage determinations. However, doxycycline is excreted primarily into the bile, and demeclocycline is metabolized in the liver.
4. Toxicity: Tetracyclines cause GI disturbances, superinfections, damage to developing teeth and bones, liver damage (particularly in pregnant women who get the drug intravenously), and photosensitization (particularly with demeclocycline). Parenteral forms are irritating.

5. Uses: These broad spectrum drugs are useful for rickettsial infections, chlamydial infections, sexually transmitted diseases, acne, and brucellosis. They have often been used as alternate therapy in penicillin-allergic patients.
6. Individual agents: The individual tetracyclines differ from one another only in the duration of their action and the stability of the drugs in the body. All are broad spectrum antibiotics.
   a. Rapidly eliminated: TETRACYCLINE (Prototype drug of this group); Oxytetracycline.
   b. More slowly eliminated: Demeclocycline and Methacycline.
   c. Long-acting: DOXYCYCLINE and Minocycline.

G. AMINOGLYCOSIDES

1. Mechanism of action: All aminoglycosides inhibit bacterial protein synthesis. Streptomycin binds to a specific site on the 30S ribosomal subunit, but other aminoglycosides bind to sites on both the 30S and 50S ribosomal subunits. The antibacterial action is usually attributed to inhibition of protein synthesis, but disruption of cell membrane function caused by transport of the antibiotics across the bacterial cell membranes may also be involved.
2. Spectrum: Aminoglycosides are bactericidal for many gram positive and gram negative bacteria. Because aminoglycosides are actively transported into a bacterial cell by an oxygen-dependent enzyme system, only aerobic bacteria are sensitive to these drugs.
3. Absorption, distribution and excretion: Aminoglycosides are not absorbed from the GI tract, but are readily absorbed from intramuscular or subcutaneous sites. They are distributed to extracellular water, but penetrate the CSF poorly, even when meninges are inflamed. They are excreted in urine after glomerular filtration of the parent compound.
4. Toxicity: Aminoglycosides cause renal toxicity, and may damage both vestibular and auditory functions of the eighth cranial nerve. Allergic reactions occasionally occur.
5. Individual agents and uses:

   a. STREPTOMYCIN - Use generally restricted to tuberculosis, bacterial endocarditis, plague, and tularemia.
   b. Neomycin - Most toxic and used only topically, or orally for gut sterilization.
   c. Kanamycin - Older agent, seldom used.
   d. GENTAMICIN, Tobramycin and Netilmicin: These agents are essentially comparable agents for systemic use in serious infections. There may be slight differences in bacterial sensitivity or potential for renal/auditory toxicity.
   e. AMIKACIN - A derivative of Kanamycin which resists inactivation by many bacterial enzymes. Many infectious disease specialists feel that amikacin should be reserved for susceptible infections resistant to other aminoglycosides.

H. FLUOROQUINOLONES (QUINOLONES)

1. Chemical class: Fluoroquinolones are chemically derived from the urinary antiseptic nalidixic acid. All are fluorinated compounds.
2. Mechanism of action: Fluoroquinolones inhibit bacterial DNA gyrase, an enzyme involved in DNA nicking and supercoiling, and are bactericidal drugs.
3. Spectrum: Fluoroquinolones are active against a wide variety of gram negative bacteria, but gram-positive organisms are usually less susceptible. Ciprofloxacin is highly active against Pseudomonas species. Anaerobic bacteria respond poorly to the fluoroquinolones.
4. Absorption, distribution and excretion: Fluoroquinolones are well-absorbed after oral administration, and are widely distributed in the body, but highest concentrations are in urine. Their relatively long-half life allows dosing twice daily. Renal excretion involves both glomerular filtration and active secretion. Fluoroquinolone metabolites have less antimicrobial activity than the parent drug.
5. Individual agents:

   CIPROFLOXACIN (oral and i.v.)   Lomefloxacin
   Norfloxacin   Enoxacin
   Ofloxacin (oral and i.v.)

6. Uses: Complicated infections of the genitourinary tract are the most common indication for fluoroquinolones. However, an important potential application is that oral fluoroquinolone therapy may replace, or shorten, some types of parenteral antibiotic therapy.
7. Toxicity: Fluoroquinolones are usually well tolerated. Irreversible damage to developing cartilage has been observed in studies with young animals, and fluoroquinolones are not recommended for patients under the age of 18.

I. SULFONAMIDES (Sulfas)---derivatives of p-aminobenzenesulfonamide

$$H_2N-\!\!\bigcirc\!\!-SO_2NHR$$

1. Mechanism of action: Sulfonamides are structurally similar to p-aminobenzoic acid (PABA), and block folic acid synthesis in microbes which must synthesize folic acid from PABA. They are bacteriostatic in concentrations which can be achieved in most body tissues and fluids, but bactericidal concentrations may be found in urine.
2. Spectrum: Sulfonamides are broad spectrum antimicrobial agents, effective against most gram positive bacteria, many gram negative bacteria, nocardia, actinomyces, chlamydia and plasmodia. Unfortunately, many strains have developed resistance to the sulfonamides.

163

3. <u>Absorption, distribution and excretion:</u> Sulfonamides are readily absorbed after oral administration. Sodium salts may be given i.v., but are strongly alkaline and cause pain and tissue sloughing if extravasated.

Sulfonamides are 20-90% bound to plasma albumin, depending on the sulfonamide and its concentration. Free (unbound) drug is distributed to total body water.

Sulfonamides are eliminated in urine by glomerular filtration and tubular secretion. Metabolites include acetylated and glucuronide conjugates, along with oxidized products.

4. <u>Toxicity:</u> Sulfonamides may precipitate in acidic urine and cause renal damage. Other adverse effects include drug allergy, toxicity to the hematopoietic system (acute hemolytic anemia, thrombocytopenia, etc.), and allergy.

5. <u>Individual agents:</u> Sulfonamides differ primarily in their pharmacokinetic properties, but are not significantly different in their antimicrobial activity.

a. <u>Short-acting sulfonamides</u>

Rapidly absorbed and excreted into urine, giving high urinary concentrations. Usually given 4 times daily.

Sulfacytine	Sulfadiazine
Sulfamethizole	Sulfisoxazole

b. <u>Intermediate-acting sulfonamide</u>

SULFAMETHOXAZOLE; longer half-life allows dosing at 8 to 12 hour intervals.

c. <u>Sulfonamide combinations</u>

1) Trisulfapyrimidines - contains equal amounts of sulfadiazine, sulfamerazine and sulfamethazine. An old "triple sulfa" formulation for additive antibacterial effects but less chance of crystalluria.
2) Sulfathiazole, sulfacetamide and sulfabenzamide - vaginal cream of questionable efficacy
3) SULFAMETHOXAZOLE AND TRIMETHOPRIM - synergistic activity of a sulfonamide plus dihydrofolate reductase inhibitor. This combination has several indications in addition to urinary tract infections.

d. <u>Miscellaneous Sulfonamides and related compounds</u>

1) Sulfacetamide - an acetylated derivative; the soluble sodium salt is widely used for ophthalmic infections.
2) Sulfapyridine - obsolete due to high risk of crystalluria, except as an alternative to dapsone for dermatitis herpetiformis.
3) Sulfasalazine - often effective in treating acute exacerbations of ulcerative colitis; however, this action is probably related to the 5-aminosalicylate portion of the molecule.

    4) Mafenide - not a true sulfonamide; used for burns.
    5) Silver sulfadiazine - less painful than mafenide and does not cause metabolic acidosis.

6. Major uses: Sulfonamides are used primarily in urinary tract infections, but have been useful in tularemia, nocardia, actinomycosis, and resistant falciparum malaria.

J. URINARY ANTISEPTICS

Urinary antiseptics are defined as substances which can be given orally, but provide significant antibacterial effects only in the urine.

1. METHENAMINE:

Dissociates into formaldehyde (the active material) and ammonia in acid urine. Bacteria do not develop resistance.

2. MANDELIC ACID:

Acidifies the urine, is antibacterial in its own right and can be added to methenamine; the mixture is known as methenamine mandelate.

3. NITROFURANTOIN:

Bactericidal activity against a number of urinary tract pathogens. The mechanism of action appears to involve bacterial metabolism of the drug, which results in the formation of reactive metabolites which attack DNA. Resistance rarely develops. Hypersensitivity reactions, nausea and vomiting are limitations to its usefulness, but a crystalline form of nitrofurantoin has a reduced incidence of gastrointestinal intolerance.

4. NALIDIXIC ACID:

Nausea, vomiting, skin rashes, and CNS effects are common; microbial resistance develops very rapidly; inhibits bacterial DNA synthesis. Cinoxacin is a chemically related drug.

5. TRIMETHOPRIM:

Selective inhibition of bacterial dihydrofolate reductase. May be bacteriostatic or bactericidal. Only approved indication as a sole agent is for uncomplicated urinary tract infections caused by susceptible organisms. Most often used in combination with sulfamethoxazole.

K. MISCELLANEOUS ANTIBACTERIAL DRUGS

1. SPECTINOMYCIN:

Spectinomycin is chemically related to the aminoglycosides. It binds at the 30S subunit of the microbial ribosome, but at a site different from that of streptomycin. The drug seems to be bacteriostatic rather than bactericidal, because of reversible binding. Spectinomycin is not absorbed orally and is given intramuscularly. It is used exclusively for one-shot treatment of gonorrhea, but is not effective against syphilis.

2. POLYMYXIN B AND COLISTIN

These are polypeptide antibiotics which are effective primarily against Gram negative organisms, particularly Pseudomonas. Renal damage and various neurological changes limit the usefulness of these drugs to topical applications. They may be used systemically in life-threatening infections resistant to safer antibiotics.

3. BACITRACIN:

Bacitracin is a polypeptide antibiotic which acts on bacterial cell walls and is effective against Gram positive organisms. Renal toxicity limits its usefulness to topical application, but it may be used in life-threatening infections which are resistant to safer antibiotics. Bacitracin is not absorbed after oral administration.

4. METRONIDAZOLE:

Metronidazole was originally developed for treatment of amebic infections, and was subsequently found to be active against many anaerobic bacteria. It is well absorbed after oral administration. It adverse effects include various neurological effects, disulfiram-like inhibition of aldehyde dehydrogenase, sodium retention, and various G.I. symptoms.

5. ANTI-TUBERCULOSIS DRUGS:

Antitubercular drugs are commonly categorized as primary or secondary agents, based on the incidence of adverse effects. The secondary (or retreatment) drugs are not as well tolerated, and are seldom used except when resistance has developed to the primary agents. Combinations of antitubercular drugs are used in therapy to decrease the incidence of bacterial resistance.

a. Primary Antitubercular Drugs:

ISONIAZID   Pyrazinamide
Ethambutol   Streptomycin
Rifampin

1) ISONIAZID (INH) is effective only against mycobacteria, and appears to affect cell wall synthesis. It can be either tuberculostatic or tuberculocidal, depending on its concentration. INH is readily absorbed after oral administration and is widely distributed in the body, including into the CSF and caseous masses. INH reacts chemically with pyridoxal and causes peripheral neuritis (adults) and convulsions (children); however, co-administration of vitamin B_6 prevents these symptoms. Otherwise, INH is usually well-tolerated. Fast acetylators metabolize the drug more rapidly than slow acetylators. INH is used for prophylaxis as well as for treatment of active infections.

2) Ethambutol is given orally, and is probably an RNA-synthesis inhibitor. Resistance develops slowly. The drug is usually well tolerated, but retrobulbar neuritis (visual field defects) is seen occasionally at high doses.

3) Rifampin (one of a family of rifamycin antibiotics) is orally effective against TB and other microbes, and inhibits DNA-directed RNA synthesis. Its usefulness is limited by rapid development of bacterial resistance.

4) Pyrazinamide is orally effective, but its mechanism of action is uncertain. Patients must be monitored for signs of hepatotoxicity.

b. Secondary Antitubercular Drugs

Aminosalicylic acid   Capreomycin
Ethionamide   Kanamycin
Cycloserine

6. ANTI-LEPROSY DRUGS

a. Dapsone (DDS) has a mechanism of action which is similar to that of sulfonamides. Its long half-life permits once-a-week administration. Hemolysis is a serious side effect, and exacerbation of lepromatous leprosy may occur. Dapsone is sometimes used in the treatment of chloroquine-resistant malaria.

b. Clofazimine has anti-inflammatory properties combined with slow antibacterial effects. Its mechanism of action is uncertain.

III. ANTIFUNGAL AGENTS

A. POLYENE ANTIFUNGALS

"Polyene" antifungals are named for large numbers of unsaturated bonds in their chemical structures. These drugs permeate into ergosterol-rich membranes (characteristic of fungi) where they produce a detergent-like effect.

1. <u>Nystatin</u> is highly toxic and is not used parenterally. It is available in a variety of preparations for topical application, and is found in tablets and suspensions for Candida infections of the mouth or GI tract. Nystatin is not absorbed after oral administration.

2. <u>Amphotericin B</u> is also not effective after oral administration, and is given by i.v. injection. It has a broad antifungal spectrum, and is useful for most systemic fungal infections. Amphotericin B causes a large number of adverse effects, but renal toxicity is the most serious. Its use is indicated only because of the seriousness of many systemic fungal infections, and marginal effectiveness of better-tolerated drugs.

B. FLUCYTOSINE

Flucytosine is effective orally for systemic Candida or Cryptococcal infections. Fungi metabolize the drug to its active form, 5-fluorouracil. Flucytosine is often used in combination with amphotericin B. Patients must be monitored carefully for hematologic, renal and hepatic function.

C. IMIDAZOLE ANTIFUNGAL AGENTS

Imidazole antifungal agents interfere with cytochrome P-450-dependent biosynthesis of ergosterol, causing disorganization of the fungal cell membrane. These agents have a broad spectrum of activity against pathogenic fungi. They may also inhibit a number of cytochrome P-450 dependent drug oxidations in patients.

1. <u>Miconazole</u> can be given intravenously in the treatment of systemic fungal infections. However, parenteral use of miconazole is associated with a rather high incidence of adverse effects, including phlebitis, pruritus, nausea and anemia.

2. <u>Ketoconazole</u> is orally effective, generally well-tolerated, and is the imidazole of choice for a variety of systemic fungal infections. The drug is only absorbed under acidic conditions, and is cleared almost exclusively by hepatic metabolism. Adverse effects include nausea, headaches, pruritus, and dizziness. Hepatic enzyme levels may be temporarily elevated, but fatal hepatic necrosis has occurred, so monitoring of liver function is necessary for long-term therapy.

3. Imidazoles which are used only topically: Clotrimazole, butoconazole, econazole, and oxiconazole.

D. TETRAZOLE ANTIFUNGAL AGENTS:

The tetrazole drugs are chemically related to imidazoles, and also act by inhibiting ergosterol biosynthesis by fungal cytochrome P-450 enzymes.

1. Fluconazole is useful for a variety of systemic fungal infections, but its penetration into the CSF makes it especially useful for Cryptoccal meningitis. Fluconazole is eliminated in the urine, and dosage modifications are necessary in cases of renal insufficiency.

2. Itraconazole is similar to ketoconazole and fluconazole in its properties and indications. Unlike fluconazole, itraconazole is cleared by hepatic metabolism.

E. GRISEOFULVIN

Griseofulvin is given orally for treatment of persistent ringworm infections, but prolonged administration is required. A variety of side effects may occur, including GI disturbances, CNS abnormalities and skin rashes.

IV. ANTIVIRAL DRUGS

A. AMANTADINE:

AMANTADINE is a highly selective antiviral drug that inhibits the growth of influenza A viruses by acting as an ion channel blocker. It is completely absorbed from the GI tract and excreted unchanged in the urine. CNS side effects (nervousness, confusion, insomnia, lightheadedness, hallucinations) are the most common. Amantadine is useful in the prophylaxis and treatment of influenza A virus infections.

B. INHIBITORS OF NUCLEIC ACID SYNTHESIS

Most inhibitors of nucleic acid synthesis are nucleoside analogs that must be phosphorylated intracellularly to exert their antiviral effects. They act by inhibiting viral replication.

1. VIDARABINE (adenine arabinoside) inhibits viral DNA polymerase; when incorporated into viral DNA, it acts as a chain terminator. A poorly soluble drug, it must be administered i.v. in large volumes of fluid. It is rapidly deaminated in liver and plasma. Adverse effects include GI disturbances, skin rash, and neurologic abnormalities (rare). Vidarabine is used to treat herpes simplex encephalitis, herpes simplex in neonates, herpes-zoster in immunosuppressed patients, and herpes simplex keratitis (topically).

2. <u>ACYCLOVIR</u> (acycloguanosine) inhibits DNA polymerase and, once incorporated into viral DNA, terminates chain elongation. Its remarkable selective toxicity depends on virus-specified thymidine kinase and viral DNA polymerase. Acyclovir is poorly absorbed by the oral route; it is excreted primarily unchanged in urine. Acyclovir is well tolerated. Indications for acyclovir include genital herpes, herpes simplex encephalitis, neonatal herpes, and herpetic infections in immunocompromized patients.

3. <u>GANCICLOVIR</u> is structurally and mechanistically similar to acyclovir. It is active against herpes viruses and is 100 times more active against cytomegalovirus than is acyclovir. Ganciclovir is administered by i.v. infusion because of poor oral absorption. Its major toxicity is bone marrow depression and its use is limited to CMV infection in immunocompromised patients.

4. <u>RIBAVIRIN</u> is a deoxyguanosine analog that contains a fraudulent base. It acts by multiple mechanisms and is effective against respiratory syncytial virus and influenza viruses (A & B). Ribavirin is administered by aerosol because of systemic toxicity (hemolytic anemic). Its use is limited to infants and children with severe, lower respiratory tract RSV.

5. <u>ZIDOVUDINE (AZT)</u> is a thymidine analog in which an azido group replaces the 3'-hydroxyl group of deoxyribose. It inhibits reverse transcriptase and causes DNA chain termination. Zidovudine is active against HIV-1 and other retroviruses. The drug is rapidly absorbed from the GI tract, metabolized to a glucuronide, and excreted into the urine. Dose-limiting toxicities are granulocytopenia and anemia; additional toxicities include severe headache, nausea, insomnia and myalgia. Zidovudine is indicated for HIV-infected adult patients with CD_4 cell counts of less than 500.

6. <u>Idoxuridine and trifluridine.</u> These analogs of thymidine act by inhibiting viral DNA polymerase. Host toxicity (bone marrow depression) is sufficient to prevent their use for systemic infections; they are used topically to treat herpes simplex keratitis.

V. ANTISEPTICS AND DISINFECTANTS

Germicides which are too toxic for internal use, but which may be effective for removal of microbes from the skin (disinfectants) or surgical instruments (antiseptics) have important roles in medicine or dentistry. These agents may be classified by their chemical nature, and some examples are given below:

A. DETERGENTS:

Anionic - ordinary soaps
Cationic - benzalkonium chloride

B. PHENOLS (Probably also act as detergents):

Phenol   Hexylresorcinol
Cresol   Hexachlorophene

C. ALCOHOLS:

Ethanol   Isopropyl alcohol

D. HALOGENS:

Chlorine   Chloramines   Iodine

E. METALS:

Silver (used in combination with sulfadiazine; see sulfonamides)
Mercury (Thimersol)

F. OXIDANTS:

Hydrogen peroxide   Permanganate
Sodium peroxide   Perborate

REVIEW QUESTIONS

ONE BEST ANSWER

1. A broad spectrum antibiotic:

   A. Isoniazid
   B. Erythromycin
   C. Doxycycline
   D. Procaine penicillin G
   E. Cefadroxil

2. A narrow spectrum antibiotic, effective only against gram-negative bacteria:

   A. Aztreonam
   B. Amikacin
   C. Chloramphenicol
   D. Sulfamethoxazole
   E. Ciprofloxacin

3. Sulbactam and tazobactam most closely resemble this drug in their antimicrobial effects:

   A. Monobactam
   B. Clindamycin
   C. Piperacillin
   D. Clavulanic acid
   E. Aztreonam

4. All of the following statements are true of both lincomycin and clindamycin **EXCEPT**:

   A. The drugs inhibit protein synthesis by binding at, or near, the ribosomal site where erythromycin binds.
   B. The antibacterial spectrum is similar to that of penicillin G and erythromycin
   C. Relatively good penetration into the bone is a beneficial feature of these antibiotics
   D. The drugs are well absorbed from the GI tract
   E. Hepatic metabolism and biliary excretion are more important than elimination by the kidneys for clearance of the drugs

5. All of the following statements are true of cephalosporins **EXCEPT**:

   A. Effectiveness against gram negative bacteria follows the order of first generation < second generation < third generation
   B. Effectiveness against gram positive bacteria follows the order of first generation < second generation < third generation
   C. Orally effective agents are available in all three generations
   D. Biliary excretion is an important route of elimination for some cephalosporins
   E. First generation cephalosporins are essentially equivalent with regard to their antibacterial effects

6. Relatively resistant to bacterial enzymes which conjugate and inactivate aminoglycosides:

   A. Amikacin
   B. Gentamicin
   C. Kanamycin
   D. Neomycin
   E. Streptomycin

7. The following drug is used only topically and for infections localized in the GI tract:

   A. Fluconazole
   B. Ketoconazole
   C. Griseofulvin
   D. Flucytosine
   E. Nystatin

8. Crystalluria and subsequent renal damage are potential adverse effects of:

   A. Amphotericin B
   B. Methenamine
   C. Neomycin
   D. Sulfadiazine
   E. Vancomycin

172

ONE BEST ANSWER

9. The following antimicrobials are indicated almost exclusively for urinary tract infections, with the exception of:

A. Methenamine
B. Sulfasalazine
C. Nalidixic acid
D. Sulfadiazine
E. Nitrofurantoin

10. An orally effective, broad spectrum antibiotic:

A. Chloramphenicol
B. Cephadroxil
C. Imipenem
D. Streptomycin
E. Clarithromycin

11. Which one of the following drugs is both orally effective and penicillinase resistant?

A. Amoxicillin
B. Carbenicillin
C. Dicloxacillin
D. Benzathine penicillin G
E. Methicillin

12. A "monobactam" antibiotic:

A. Sulbactam
B. Vancomycin
C. Spectinomycin
D. Aztreonam
E. Loracarbef

13. Combinations of antibiotics are sometimes used together to achieve synergistic antibacterial effects. Which one of the following combinations are synergistic because they affect a common bacterial biosynthetic pathway at two different points?

A. Ampicillin plus gentamicin
B. Clavulanic acid plus amoxicillin
C. Tetracycline plus penicillin V
D. Sulfamethoxazole plus trimethoprim
E. Methenamine plus mandelic acid

14 Very long half-life is related to its accumulation in tissues:

A. Azithromycin
B. Aztreonam
C. Doxycycline
D. Chloramphenicol
E. Sulfamethoxazole

15. Lethal synthesis is the activation of drugs to metabolites which produce selective toxic effects. All of the drugs below undergo lethal synthesis EXCEPT:

A. Acyclovir
B. Cytarabine
C. Zidovudine
D. Amantadine
E. Mercaptopurine

16. Which one of the following drugs has the greatest selective toxicity against herpes simplex virus?

A. Vidarabine
B. Idoxuridine
C. Ribavirin
D. Acyclovir
E. Amantadine

17. Which one of the following drugs is used to treat respiratory syncytial virus?

A. Interferon
B. Ribavirin
C. Vidarabine
D. Rimantadine
E. Acyclovir

18. Which one of the following agents is used for topical treatment of herpes simplex keratitis?

A. Idoxuridine
B. Interferon gamma
C. Amantadine
D. Ribavirin
E. Zidovudine

173

ONE BEST ANSWER

19. Which one of the following antiviral agents inhibits reverse transcriptase?

A. Acyclovir
B. Amantadine
C. Idoxuridine
D. Zidovudine
E. Vidarabine

20. Which one of the following is the major toxicity of zidovudine?

A. Bone marrow depression
B. Renal failure
C. Flu-like syndrome
D. Convulsions
E. Hepatotoxicity

21. Amantadine:

A. Is not absorbed orally
B. Is rapidly glucuronidated in the liver
C. Blocks the penetration of vaccinia virus into the cell
D. Can cause nervousness, insomnia, hallucinations, seizures
E. Is indicated for treatment of influenza B virus infections

MATCHING: Use a letter only once.
Match each of the following chemotherapeutic agents with its probable mechanism of action:

Mechanisms: Metabolic function inhibited:

A. Cell wall synthesis: interaction with penicillin binding proteins
B. Cell wall synthesis: transport of precursor units
C. Cell membrane: detergent-like effect
D. Cell membrane: inhibits sterol biosynthesis
E. Protein synthesis: 30S ribosomal subunit
F. Protein synthesis: 50S ribosomal subunit
G. Nucleic acids: inhibition of polymerase
H. Nucleic acids: inhibition of DNA gyrase
I. Nucleic acids: intercalation of DNA
J. Nucleic acids: antimetabolite causes inhibition of DNA synthesis
K. Nucleic acids: alkylation of DNA

Drugs:

22. Doxycycline

23. Zidovudine

24. Imipenem

25. Benzalkonium chloride

26. Cyclophosphamide

27. Fluconazole

28. Sulfamethoxazole

29. Vancomycin

30. Ofloxacin

31. Azithromycin

32. Doxorubicin

MATCHING: Use a letter only once.

For each of the disease states listed below, pick the antimicrobial agent which would most likely be indicated:

A. Penicillin G   G. Dicloxacillin
B. Clindamycin   H. Ceftazidime
C. Tetracycline   I. Dapsone
D. Chloramphenicol   J. Vancomycin
E. Rifampin   K. Spectinomycin
F. Clarithromycin   L. Fluconazole

Infectious diseases:

33. Rocky Mountain Spotted Fever

34. Salmonella infection

35. Cryptococcal meningitis

36. Legionnaire's Disease

37. Probable Staphylococcal infection (prior to sensitivity testing)

38. Leprosy

39. Systemic infection of Pseudomonas aeruginosa

40. Gonorrhea (single dose treatment)

41. Tuberculosis

42. Bacteroides fragilis infection

43. Methicillin-resistant staphylococcal infection

MATCHING: Use a letter only once.

Antifungal Drugs:

A. Amphotericin B
B. Flucytosine
C. Griseofulvin
D. Itraconazole
E. Ketoconazole

Descriptions:

44. A fungistatic drug which is given orally for persistent infections of the skin and nails.

45. A broad spectrum tetrazole which is eliminated by hepatic metabolism

46. Direct detergent-like effect on fungal membranes

47. Potential drug interaction with antacids because an acidic pH is required for its absorption from the GI tract

48. An inactive "pro-drug", which is converted to its active metabolite by fungal enzymes, but not mammalian enzymes

MATCHING: Use a letter only once.

Match the antibiotic listed below with the toxicity most commonly attributed to it.

A. Ciprofloxacin
B. Metronidazole
C. Gentamicin
D. Erythromycin estolate
E. Chloramphenicol

Adverse Effects:

49. Disulfiram-like effects

50. Cholestatic jaundice

51. Damage to developing cartilage

52. Aplastic anemia

53. Vestibular toxicity

CHAPTER 10: CANCER CHEMOTHERAPY AND IMMUNOSUPPRESSIVE AGENTS

I. CANCER CHEMOTHERAPY

A. GENERAL

A number of neoplastic diseases can be cured with drugs alone or with drugs in combination with other modalities (e.g., choriocarcinoma, Hodgkin's disease, acute leukemia, Burkitt's lymphoma, testicular carcinoma). Adjuvant chemotherapy in combination with surgery and/or radiotherapy has increased survival rates for a number of solid tumors. However, the most prevalent forms of human cancer respond poorly or not at all to chemotherapy.

Cancer chemotherapeutic agents generally have low therapeutic indices and potentially lethal toxicities. Many of the toxic effects of anticancer drugs are due to cytotoxic effects on normal tissues which have high proportions of dividing cells. These tissues include the bone marrow (cytopenias, increased risk of infection or activation of latent infection, immunosuppression, hemorrhage), digestive tract (oral and/or intestinal ulceration, diarrhea), hair root (alopecia), gonads (menstrual irregularities, amenorrhea, infertility, impaired spermatogenesis, sterility), repairing tissues (impaired healing) and fetus (teratogenesis). Anticancer drugs frequently produce nausea and vomiting which can be ameliorated with phenothiazines or cannabinoids. The release of nucleic acid breakdown products following a very large cell kill can result in hyperuricemia and renal damage; hyperuricemia is prevented with allopurinol. Many anticancer drugs are mutagenic and carcinogenic.

An understanding of cell kinetics is essential for the proper use of anticancer agents. Most anticancer drugs kill dividing cells (are proliferation dependent); thus, tumors with a high growth fraction are most susceptible (certain leukemias and lymphomas, small proliferating tumors, "recruited" tumor cells, micrometastases). The killing of tumor cells follows first order kinetics. To produce a cure, therapy must continue until the last tumor cell is gone. Agents which act preferentially on tumor cells in a given phase of the cell cycle are called cycle phase specific. Some agents act during several stages of the cell cycle, are nonspecific. Optimal scheduling is important.

Cancer chemotherapy usually involves a combination of drugs. Ideally, drugs are selected which are effective when used alone, and have different mechanisms of action, minimally overlapping toxicities and no cross resistance. Doses close to the regular doses for each drug as a single agent can be used to optimize the cytotoxic effects without getting additive toxicity; the development of drug resistance is diminished. Drug resistance is the greatest obstacle to successful chemotherapy.

B. ALKYLATING AGENTS

These drugs bind covalently to DNA and other cell constituents, DNA cross-linking produces cytotoxicity, main result is inhibition of DNA replication and transcription; proliferation dependent, cycle phase nonspecific. High rates of DNA repair may be a cause of resistance. Bone marrow depression is the major toxicity for all of the alkylating agents.

1. <u>MECHLORETHAMINE</u>: first anticancer drug to be used clinically; better-tolerated drugs are more often used today; i.v.; highly-reactive; potent vesicant; bone-marrow depression is dose-limiting; severe nausea and vomiting. Main use is in MOPP regimen.
2. <u>CYCLOPHOSPHAMIDE</u>: Most widely used alkylating agent; requires cytochrome P450- mediated metabolism for activation; nonvesicant; oral or i.v.; bone marrow depression is dose-limiting; alopecia and immunosuppression are prominent; sterile hemorrhagic cystitis is preventable with adequate hydration.
3. <u>MELPHALAN</u>: phenylalanine derivative of mechlorethamine; effective orally; provides gradual but continuous administration. Its mechanism of action and its toxicity are similar to that of the other alkylating agents. Drug of choice for multiple myeloma.
4. <u>Nitrosoureas (carmustine, lomustine)</u>: Bind through an alkyl or a carbamoyl moiety; are highly lipophilic and cross the blood-brain barrier; used to treat CNS malignancies; bone marrow depression is <u>delayed</u> and may be prolonged.
5. <u>Busulfan</u>: Bone marrow depression is selective for granulocytes; used to treat chronic granulocytic leukemia; leukopenia; skin pigmentation.
6. <u>Procarbazine</u>: Must undergo metabolic activation; several mechanisms of action possible; not cross resistant with other alkylating agents; oral; bone marrow depression is dose-limiting; CNS depression (synergistic with phenothiazines, barbiturates).

C. ANTIMETABOLITES

Act primarily by inhibiting DNA synthesis; inhibit cells in S-phase (except fluorouracil which has no clear-cut phase specificity); may be incorporated into DNA and RNA; major toxicity is bone marrow depression. The purine and pyrimidine analogs require "lethal synthesis" for activity.

1. <u>METHOTREXATE</u>: Folic acid analogue, competitively inhibits dihydrofolate reductase; oral, i.v., intrathecal; 50% bound to plasma proteins (displaced by salicylates, sulfonamides, etc.); excreted unchanged in urine (caution in patients with renal damage); is sometimes used in very high doses with leucovorin rescue; oral and GI ulceration, bone marrow depression are dose-limiting toxicities; hepatic and renal damage; drug of choice for gestational choriocarcinoma; also used for psoriasis and rheumatoid arthritis.

2. <u>MERCAPTOPURINE</u>: Purine analog, major mechanisms of action are psuedofeedback inhibition of the first step in purine biosynthesis and inhibition of purine interconversions; oral; metabolism to inactive products is inhibited by allopurinol; bone marrow depression is major toxicity; liver damage.
3. <u>THIOGUANINE</u>: Like mercaptopurine EXCEPT allopurinol does not interfere with its inactivation.
4. <u>FLUOROURACIL</u>: Pyrimidine analogue, cytotoxicity is associated with inhibition of thymidylate synthesis and incorporation into RNA; <u>no</u> cycle phase specificity; i.v.; rapidly metabolized in liver, enters CSF; oral and GI ulcers, bone marrow depression are dose-limiting; neurological defects (cerebellar); hyperpigmentation, alopecia.
5. <u>Cytarabine</u>: A pyrimidine nucleoside analogue (cytosine arabinoside); inhibits DNA synthesis by becoming incorporated into DNA with subsequent defects in elongation; i.v., rapidly deaminated in liver, plasma, and other tissues; bone marrow depression is major toxicity; oral ulceration, hepatic dysfunction.

D. ANTIBIOTICS

So called because they are isolated from different species of <u>Streptomyces</u>; act by binding to DNA (noncovalently, by intercalation) and altering its function; cycle phase nonspecific; bone marrow depression is the major toxicity, EXCEPT for bleomycin.

1. <u>DACTINOMYCIN (Actinomycin D)</u>: Intercalates between G-C pairs in double-stranded DNA, inhibits DNA-directed RNA synthesis; equally cytotoxic to proliferating and stationary cells; i.v., local inflammation and phlebitis; bone marrow toxicity is dose limiting; oral and GI ulceration, alopecia.
2. <u>DOXORUBICIN (Adriamycin)</u>: Possible mechanisms of action include: inhibition of DNA and RNA synthesis due to intercalation, DNA fragmentation from reactive oxygen species, inhibition of DNA topoisomerase II, and interaction with cell membranes; broad spectrum of antitumor activity; i.v., extravasation leads to severe local reaction and necrosis, extensively metabolized in liver and excreted into bile (decrease dose in presence of hepatic dysfunction); drug and metabolites color urine red. Bone marrow depression is dose-limiting; <u>cardiotoxicity</u> (refractory congestive heart failure) is due to avid uptake by and oxidative damage to heart muscle, is delayed many months, is related to total dose administered, may be irreversible. Other toxicities: alopecia, stomatitis, fever and chills.
3. <u>DAUNORUBICIN</u>: like doxorubicin EXCEPT narrower spectrum of activity.
4. <u>Plicamycin (Mithramycin)</u>: Inhibits DNA-directed RNA synthesis; i.v.; is highly toxic; produces hemorrhagic diathesis and bone marrow depression. Used in lower doses to treat hypercalcemia.
5. <u>BLEOMYCIN</u>: A mixture of complex glycopeptides; causes strand scission of DNA by producing reactive oxygen species; is unusual in that it produces very little bone marrow depression; i.v.; is enzymatically inactivated in a number of tissues, toxicity occurs in tissues with low inactivating activity, 50% is excreted

unchanged in urine; pulmonary toxicity (pneumonitis and fibrosis) is dose-limiting; most common toxic effects involve skin and mucous membranes; other toxicities: alopecia, stomatitis.

E. ANTIMITOTICS

Bind to tubulin, inhibit mitotic spindles, arrest cells in M phase; given i.v. (extravasation and local reaction); excreted into bile (caution in patients with obstructive jaundice). The vinca alkaloids, vincristine and vinblastine, are structurally similar but have different activities and toxicities, and no cross-resistance.

1. VINCRISTINE: Neurological toxicities are dose-limiting, suppression of achilles tendon reflex and paresthesias appear first, followed by other peripheral neuropathies, neuritic pain, constipation, disorders of cranial nerve function; alopecia; mild bone marrow depression. Vincristine is considered to be marrow sparing compared to other agents.
2. VINBLASTINE: Bone marrow depression is dose-limiting; other toxicities: alopecia, stomatitis, peripheral neuropathy. Neuropathy is less frequent and less serious than with vincristine.

F. HORMONES AND HORMONE INHIBITORS

Hormonal therapy in the form of ablation is effective for some cancers; in breast cancer, demonstration of the presence of estrogen receptors identifies those tumors most likely to respond to hormonal therapy. The use of hormones is largely empirical; they may inhibit tumor growth directly or oppose the effects of endogenous hormones. Toxicities are due to hormonal effects rather than cytotoxic effects.

1. Corticosteroids (PREDNISONE): Lympholytic; used in combination with other agents to treat lymphomatous cancers; are not myelosuppressive; psychoses and euphoria, gastric ulcers, glucose intolerance, osteoporosis, cataract formation, sodium and water retention, immunosuppressive.
2. Estrogens: used in breast cancer, prostate cancer; nausea and vomiting, fluid retention, hypercalcemia; gynecomastia, impotence; cardiovascular complications with larger doses.
3. Antiestrogen (TAMOXIFEN): Competitive antagonist of estrogen, may inhibit replication by additional mechanisms; used in breast cancer; nausea and vomiting, hot flashes, hypercalcemia.
4. LEUPROLIDE: A GnRH agonist; desensitizes pituitary GnRH receptors and inhibits gonadotropin release; used in prostate cancer. Combined use with antiandrogen (e.g., flutamide) prevents initial flare-up of disease. Hot flashes are common; other side effects: gynecomastia, nausea and vomiting, edema, thrombophlebitis.

H. MISCELLANEOUS

1. CISPLATIN: A platinum coordination complex, probably acts by forming DNA cross-links; i.v., 90% bound to plasma proteins, concentrates in liver, kidney, intestines and ovary; excreted in urine; renal damage is dose-limiting (is decreased by prehydration and concomitant mannitol diuresis); other toxicities: moderate bone marrow depression, ototoxicity, hypomagnesemia and hypocalcemia.
2. ETOPOSIDE: Inhibits DNA topoisomerase II; leukopenia is dose-limiting, other toxicities include alopecia, stomatitis, nausea and vomiting.
3. Interferon alpha 2 is approved for use in the treatment of hairy cell leukemia and for condylomata acuminata (genital warts); usually administered i.m.; degraded in kidney; fever, chills, myalgia, fatigue, and weakness occur in most patients.

II.   IMMUNOSUPPRESSIVE AGENTS

A. CYCLOSPORINE: Cyclic undecapeptide; prevents cytotoxic T lymphocyte activation at an early stage; oral or i.v., 90% bound, fully metabolized; prophylaxis of organ rejection; major toxicity is renal, others: hepatotoxicity, increased susceptibility to infection and development of lymphomas.
B. Azathioprine: Similar to mercaptopurine but greater immunosuppressive activity.
C. Anticancer drugs: Cyclophosphamide, methotrexate, others.
D. Glucocorticoids: Prednisone, others.

III.   STUDY AIDE

The table below summarizes the major mechanism of action and dose-limiting toxicity for each group of cancer chemotherapeutic drugs. Fill in one or two distinguishing characteristic(s) for each individual agent. Some examples are given.

DRUG	ACTION	TOXICITY
Alkylating agents:	Bind covalently to DNA; inhibit DNA synthesis; cycle phase nonspecific	Bone marrow depression
Busulfan		
Cyclophosphamide	Reqs. activ. by cyt P-450;	Hemorrhagic cystitis
Mechlorethamine		
Melphalan		
Nitrosoureas		
Procarbazine		

Antimetabolites:	Inhibit DNA synthesis; S-phase specific (except 5-FU); require lethal synth. (except MTX)	Bone marrow depression, oral and GI ulceration, (hepatotoxicity)
Cytarabine		
Fluorouracil		
Mercaptopurine	Reduce dose with allopurinol	
Methotrexate		
Thioguanine		

DRUG	ACTION	TOXICITY
Antibiotics:	Bind to DNA by intercalation, inhibit DNA or RNA synth.; cycle phase nonspecific	Bone marrow depression (except BLEO)
Bleomycin		Pulmonary toxicity, cutaneous reactions
Dactinomycin		
Daunorubicin		
Doxorubicin (Adriamycin)		
Plicamycin	Used for hypercalcemia	Hemorrhagic diathesis
Antimitotics:	Bind to tubulin, inhibit mitotic spindles, M-phase specific	Bone marrow depression, neurotoxicity
Vinblastine		
Vincristine		
Hormones:	Alter hormonal environm., mainly palliative	Fluid retention, hypercalcemia is common
Estrogens		
Corticosteroids		
Antiestrogens		
Leuprolide		
Miscellaneous:		
Cisplatin:	Crosslinks DNA	Renal damage, bone marrow depression, ototoxicity
Etoposide:	Inhibits DNA topoisomerase	Bone marrow depression
Interferon alpha		Flu-like syndrome

182

REVIEW QUESTIONS

ONE BEST ANSWER

1. An antitumor drug with selective toxicity for the granulocytic series of white blood cells is:

   A. Mercaptopurine
   B. Mechlorethamine
   C. Cyclosporin
   D. Busulfan
   E. Prednisone

2. An analog of mercaptopurine that is used as an immunosuppressant in allotransplantation procedures:

   A. Azathioprine
   B. Allopurinol
   C. Cisplatin
   D. Mechlorethamine
   E. Busulfan

3. Leucovorin is used to "rescue" normal cells after massive doses of:

   A. Mechlorethamine
   B. Dactinomycin
   C. Fluorouracil
   D. Methotrexate
   E. Mercaptopurine

4. Drugs used as immunosuppressive agents include all of the following **EXCEPT**:

   A. Cyclosporin
   B. Mechlorethamine
   C. Azathioprine
   D. Cyclophosphamide
   E. Prednisone

5. Which one of the following drugs acts by inhibiting DNA topoisomerase?

   A. Cyclophosphamide
   B. Methotrexate
   C. Etoposide
   D. Leuprolide
   E. Fluorouracil

6. Which one of the following is NOT one of the guidelines used in selecting drugs for combination chemotherapy?

   A. Each drug should be active against the tumor when used alone
   B. Each drug should exhibit cycle phase specificity
   C. The drugs should act by different mechanisms
   D. The drugs should be optimally scheduled
   E. The drugs should have minimally overlapping toxicities

7. Mucocutaneous changes (hyperpigmentation, pruritic erythema, hyperkeratosis, desquamation, mucositis) occur frequently with:

   A. Daunorubicin
   B. Cyclophosphamide
   C. Prednisone
   D. Bleomycin
   E. Vinblastine

8. Which one of the following statements is true of melphalan but not true of mechlorethamine?

   A. Forms covalent bonds with DNA
   B. Is administered by the oral route
   C. Causes bone marrow depression
   D. Cytotoxicity is related to DNA cross-linking
   E. Increased rates of DNA repair may cause resistance

183

MATCHING: Use a letter only once

   A. Vincristine
   B. Cyclophosphamide
   C. Doxorubicin
   D. Mercaptopurine
   E. Tamoxifen

9. Inhibition of purine biosynthesis

10. Intercalation with DNA

11. Inhibition of mitotic spindles

12. Alkylation of DNA

13. Inhibition of estrogen

MATCHING: Use a letter only once

   A. Vincristine
   B. Leuprolide
   C. Daunorubicin
   D. Bleomycin
   E. Carmustine

18. Cardiotoxicity

19. Hot flashes

20. Pneumonitis

21. Neurotoxicity

22. Delayed bone marrow depression

MATCHING: Use a letter only once

   A. Mercaptopurine
   B. Vinblastine
   C. Doxorubicin
   D. Methotrexate

14. Lower dosage required in patients with impaired renal excretion

15. Lower dosage required when patient is also taking allopurinol

16. Lower cumulative dose in patients who have had radiotherapy to the heart

17. Lower dosage in patients with impaired liver function

CHAPTER 11: <u>CHEMOTHERAPY OF PARASITIC DISEASES</u>

I. **PROTOZOAN INFECTIONS**

    A. **AMEBICIDAL DRUGS** (*Entamoeba histolytica*)

        1. <u>Metronidazole</u>: Agent of choice for systemic and intestinal forms of amebiasis <u>except</u> for asymptomatic cyst carriers; also useful for trichomoniasis and lambliasis. It has a direct amebicidal effect and acts by inhibiting a unique electron transfer system of a variety of anaerobic organisms. It is orally effective and is given in combination with diloxanide to produce cures. Adverse effects include nausea, vomiting, and headache. Seizures, ataxia, leukopenia, and alcohol intolerance (disulfiram-like reaction) have been reported. Shod be avoided during pregnancy.

        2. <u>Diloxanide furoate</u>: The agent of choice in treating <u>asymptomatic cyst carrier</u> and can yield cures. Acts only in the gut lumen and when given alone is ineffective against hepatic abscess. It is inexpensive and apparently lacks serious side effects in man - flatulence is common.

        3. <u>ALTERNATE DRUGS</u>:

            a. <u>Iodoquinol</u> (Di-iodohydroxyquine)
                Directly amebicidal to trophozoites and cysts and only used for intestinal amebiasis. GI, neurotoxic effects and thyroid enlargement have been reported.

            b. <u>Emetine - dehydroemetine</u>
                Used for acute amebic dysentery and extraintestinal forms in combination with chloroquine. Directly cidal to trophozoites but not effective on cysts. GI irritation and cardiac toxicity are common.

            c. <u>Chloroquine</u>
                Useful for hepatic amebiasis only when metronidazole therapy is not successful; ineffective for intestinal amebiasis. (See section on antimalarial drugs for additional comments on chloroquine).

            d. <u>Paromomycin</u>
                Poorly absorbed aminoglycoside antibiotic; in addition to eliminating intestinal bacteria, paromomycin directly kills trophozoites and can be used to treat mild intestinal disease. It also kills intestinal cestodes.

    B. **GIARDIASIS** (*Giardia lamblia*): Metronidazole is the drug of choice with quinacrine the alternative therapy.

    C. **LEISHMANIASIS** (*Leishmania braziliensis, L. mexicana* and other species): Sodium stibogluconate, a pentavalent antimonial, is considered the drug of choice for the treatment of leishmaniasis, transmitted by sand flies. This was a Desert Storm problem and investigational new drugs are under development.

THERAPEUTIC REGIMENS FOR AMEBIASIS

	Drug of Choice	Alternates
Asymptomatic cyst passer (intestinal cysts)	Diloxanide	Iodoquinol
Mild intestinal disease (intestinal trophozoites)	Metronidazole followed by Diloxanide	Diloxanide followed by Chloroquine
Severe intestinal disease	Metronidazole followed by Diloxanide	Dehydroemetine followed by Iodoquinol
Extraintestinal disease (hepatic abscess)	Metronidazole followed by Diloxanide	Dehydroemetine followed by Chloroquine and Iodoquinol

D. ANTIMALARIAL DRUGS

Plasmodium vivax, P. ovale and P. malariae: All have erythrocytic and tissue cycles.

Plasmodium falciparum: Has no tissue (exoerythrocytic) cycle

1. Chloroquine kills erythrocytic forms but is not effective on liver forms. It is rapidly and almost completely absorbed after oral administration. It accumulates in the liver (which suggested its use for hepatic amebiasis) and is slowly excreted. Toxicity is dose related, ranging from GI distress, rashes and headache to ocular toxicity (retinopathy and corneal deposits which suggest a "bulls-eye") and CNS hyperexcitability. Methemoglobinemia and hemolytic anemia can occur in individuals with a genetic deficiency of G-6-PD. Also has anti-inflammatory effect.

2. Primaquine can destroy exo-erythrocytic, liver-lurking forms and is gametocidal. It is rapidly absorbed after oral administration and is metabolized to active forms by the liver. Mild toxicity includes anorexia, nausea, vomiting, cramps. In individuals with G-6-PD deficiency, methemoglobinemia and hemolytic anemia can occur.

3. Quinine is a traditional agent now largely replaced by newer drugs but is still useful in drug-resistant strains of *P. falciparum*. It is only effective against erythrocytic forms and not on liver forms. Toxicity: cinchonism (headache, tinnitus, diploplia); allergic skin rashes; hypotension, myocardial and skeletal muscle depression, and renal damage. It can cause intravascular hemolysis in sensitized individuals and also methemoglobinemia and hemolytic anemia in individuals with G-6-PD deficiency. All quinone antimalarials ("QUINES") possess this genetically determined toxicity.

4. DIHYDROFOLATE REDUCTASE INHIBITORS (DHRI):

Pyrimethamine is the most potent and has the longest duration of action. Chloroguanide is a pro-drug (active metabolite - cycloguanil); shortest action. Trimethoprim

- All compounds act by inhibiting dihydrofolic acid reductase and prevent the production of tetrahydrofolic acid. Resistance to one usually confers resistance to the other.
- All drugs can cause weak inhibition of human dihydrofolic acid reductase, which results in megaloblastic anemia. Folinic acid will remedy the anemia without interfering with the chemotherapy.
- All drugs act slowly. Erythrocytic and exoerythrocytic forms are inhibited.
- Use limited primarily to treatment of chloroquine-resistant *P. falciparum* but many strains are now resistant to DHRI, as well.
- Recently a combination of pyrimethamine + sulfadoxine used to treat chloroquine resistant *P. falciparum* (blocking 2 steps in folic acid synthesis).
5. Mefloquine is an antimalarial developed for treatment and prevention of chloroquine resistant *P. falciparum*. Well absorbed; well tolerated.
6. Quinacrine is an old antimalarial agent now used primarily for tapeworms or as an alternative to metronidazole for giardiasis; skin may be stained yellow.

E. PNEUMOCYSTOSIS (*Pneumocystis carinii*)

1. Trimethoprim + sulfamethoxazole, given in combination, is considered the treatment of choice for pneumocystosis.
2. Atovaquone recently was approved for the treatment of *P. Carinii* pneumonia in AIDS patients. It is effective and has relatively little toxicity.
3. Pentamidine in aerosol form is effective for the treatment of *P. Carinii* pneumonia in AIDS patients but is toxic. Given i.m., it also is effective but even more toxic when used to treat trypanosomiasis or leishmaniasis.

F. TRICHOMONIASIS (*Trichomonas vaginalis*)

Metronidazole is the drug of choice for treatment of this sexually transmitted protozoan infection.

G. TOXOPLASMOSIS

Pyrimethamine + sulfadiazine are effective against this common parasitic disease caused by *Toxoplasma gondii* .(Cats are hosts for the sexual forms).

H. TRYPANOSOMIASIS

<u>Nifurtimox</u> is the drug of choice in S. American trypanosomiasis (Chagas' disease) <u>Melarsoprol</u> (an organic arsenical) is the drug of choice for African sleeping sickness. <u>Suramin</u> and <u>pentamidine</u> also are used for the various forms.

II. METAZOAN INFECTIONS

A. NEMATODE INFECTIONS (Roundworm)

	Drug of Choice	Alternate Therapy
Roundworm (*Ascaris lumbricoides*)	Mebendazole	Pyrantel Piperazine
Pinworm (*Enterobius vermicularis*)	Mebendazole	Pyrantel Piperazine
Hookworm (*Necator americanus*) and (*Ancylostoma duodenale*)	Mebendazole	Pyrantel
Threadworm (*Strongyloides stercoralis*)	Thiabendazole	Ivermectin
Trichinosis (*Trichinella spiralis*)	Thiabendazole	Mebendazole
Whipworm (*Trichuris trichiura*)	Mebendazole	Thiabendazole

1. <u>Mebendazole</u>: Mostly unabsorbed. Binds to and inhibits tubulin synthesis; Inhibits glucose uptake and larval development. Few side effects: occasional abdominal distress and diarrhea. Contraindicated in pregnancy and drug allergies.

2. <u>Pyrantel</u>: Noncompetitive depolarizing neuromuscular block; worm paralyzed. Some mild and transient G.I., CNS, skin, and hepatic reactions.

3. Thiabendazole: Rapidly absorbed; larvicidal for cutaneous larvae migrans. Frequent mild, transient side effects (vomiting, nausea, lethargy, dizziness) reduced by giving after meals. Hepatotoxic higher doses diminish mental alertness.

4. Piperazine: Produces competitive block of ACh on worm muscle; worms are paralyzed and eliminated alive; well absorbed; mild transient G.I. effects and rash.

5. Ivermectin: New drug; paralyzes worm by actions on GABA synapses in periphery.

B. CESTODE INFECTIONS (Flatworm)

	Drug of Choice	Alternate Therapy
Beef tapeworm (*Taenia saginata*)	Praziquantel	Niclosamide
Pork tapeworm (*Taenia solium*)		
Fish tapeworm (*Diphyllobothrium latum*)	Praziquantel	Niclosamide
Dwarf tapeworm (*Hymenolepiasis nana*)	Praziquantel	Niclosamide

1. Praziquantel: New broad-spectrum anthelminthic effective for a variety of cestode and trematode infections. Well absorbed; well tolerated; no major adverse effects have been reported; increases permeability of cell membrane to Ca^{++}, causing spastic paralysis of worm muscle, followed by disintegration of its tegument.

2. Niclosamide: Not absorbed. Inhibits oxidative phosphorylation and glucose uptake. Infrequent, mild G.I. upset.
(NOTE: *Taenia solium* cysticercosis: Use antiemetics and post-therapy purgation).

C. TREMATODE INFECTIONS (Fluke)

	Drug of Choice	Alternate Therapy
Schistosomiasis (Blood fluke)	Praziquantel	---
Fasciolopsis (Intestinal fluke)	Praziquantel	---
Clonorchis and *Fasciola hepatica* (Liver fluke)	Praziquantel	---
Paragonimus (Lung fluke)	Praziquantel	---

REVIEW QUESTIONS

ONE BEST ANSWER

1. Which one of the following is the drug of choice in the treatment of amebic hepatic abscess?

   A. Emetine
   B. Metronidazole
   C. Chloroquine
   D. Iodoquinol
   E. Oxytetracycline

2. All of the following are effective against intestinal amebiasis **EXCEPT**:

   A. Metronidazole
   B. Chloroquine
   C. Iodoquinol
   D. Paromomycin
   E. Diloxanide furoate

3. Which one of the following is the drug of choice in acute amebic dysentery?

   A. Chloroquine
   B. Iodoquinol
   C. Dehydroemetine
   D. Metronidazole
   E. Diloxanide furoate

4. Which one of the following is the drug of choice in the treatment of asymptomatic amebic cyst carriers?

   A. Emetine
   B. Iodoquinol
   C. Diloxanide furoate
   D. Metronidazole

5. Which one of the following drugs would be most effective in producing a radical cure of a Plasmodium vivax infection?

   A. Chloroquine
   B. Pyrimethamine
   C. Primaquine
   D. Quinacrine
   E. Quinidine

6. Which one of the following mechanisms best accounts for the schizonticidal effect of pyrimethamine?

   A. Inhibition of mitochondrial oxidative phosphorylation
   B. Inhibition of dihydrofolate reductase
   C. Competition with para-aminobenzoic acid in the synthesis of folic acid
   D. Intercalation between the strands of DNA thus inhibiting DNA polymerase
   E. Decrease in glucose uptake by the parasite

7. Which one of the following drugs has cross-resistance with pyrimethamine?

   A. Quinine
   B. Quinacrine
   C. Chloroquine
   D. Chloroguanide
   E. Primaquine

8. A drug effective for the treatment of pork tapeworm (Taenia solium) infestation is:

   A. Thiabendazole
   B. Bephenium
   C. Pyrivinium
   D. Praziquantil
   E. Piperazine

9. A drug effective for the treatment of pinworm (ENTEROBIASIS) infestation is:

   A. Niridazole
   B. Bephenium
   C. Niclosamide
   D. Mebendazole
   E. Chloroquine

10. Which of the following drugs is effective in a single oral dose against roundworm and pinworm infestation?

    A. Bephenium
    B. Stibophen
    C. Mebendazole
    D. Diethylcarbamazine
    E. Niridazole

ONE BEST ANSWER

11. A drug effective in the treatment of hookworm infestations is:

A. Praziquantil
B. Iodoquinol
C. Piperazine
D. Niridazole
E. Mebendazole

12. All of the following are true of mebendazole **EXCEPT**:

A. Irreversibly inhibits helminthic glucose uptake
B. Is contraindicated in pregnancy
C. Is a broad spectrum agent effective against intestinal nematodes
D. Has few adverse effects
E. Is completely absorbed after oral administration

13. Chloroquine:

A. Is not absorbed
B. Can cause retinopathy (the bull's eye lesion)
C. Acts against hepatic plasmodial forms
D. Effective against intestinal trophozoites in amebiasis
E. Does not bind and accumulate in tissue

14. All of the following are true of primaquine **EXCEPT**:

A. Rapidly absorbed after oral administration
B. Has some metabolites with greater antimalarial activity than the parent compound
C. Can cause hemolytic anemia in susceptible individuals
D. Acts by inhibiting dihydrofolic acid reductase
E. Has gametocidal action

CHAPTER 12: <u>GASTROINTESTINAL DRUGS</u>

I. UPPER GI DISORDERS

A. DRUG TREATMENT OF PEPTIC ULCERS

Recent studies have provided a growing body of evidence that the microorganism Helicobacter pylori plays a major role in the etiology of ulcer disease and gastritis and possibly even gastric carcinoma. Some mysteries remain to be solved regarding the etiology of ulcer disease. The older anti-ulcer agents which have been used successfully in the past should not be abandoned as the indiscriminate use of antibiotics in therapy could promote the development of antibiotic-resistant strains of the bacterium. Clinical trials are being conducted to establish therapeutic guidelines for therapy of ulcer disease in the future.

1. HISTAMINE (H_2) RECEPTOR ANTAGONISTS

These drugs act specifically to block competitively the H_2 histamine receptors of parietal cells. They inhibit gastric acid secretion, both basal and stimulated secretion. They promote the healing of duodenal ulcer and also have proved useful in the treatment of reflux esophagitis, Zollinger-Ellison syndrome and systemic mastocytosis.

<u>Cimetidine</u>: Adverse effects include headache, nausea and skin rash. It binds to androgen receptors and gynecomastia and impotence may occur. It inhibits drug metabolizing enzymes, possibly leading to drug interactions. Rarely it has been reported to cause agranulocytosis and thrombocytopenia.

<u>Ranitidine</u>: Is 5 to 10x more potent and has a longer duration of action. It lacks the enzyme inhibitory and androgenic effects seen with cimetidine. The incidence of adverse effects, such as headaches and rash, is low.

<u>Famitodine</u>: Approximately twice as potent as ranitidine and can be given once daily. Side effects are similar.

<u>Nizatidine</u>: The newest of these agents also can be given once daily.

2. H^+-K^+-ATPase (PROTON PUMP) INHIBITORS

<u>Omeprazole</u>: The first of a new class of agents. It inhibits the proton pump of the parietal cells of the stomach, thus inhibiting acid secretion.
Orally effective agent with minimal adverse effects. Recently also approved for the treatment of reflux esophagitis.

3. GASTRIC ANTACIDS

These agents are weak bases which can neutralize the hydrochloric acid secreted by the parietal cells of the stomach. They are used in the therapy of peptic ulcer or hyperchlorhydria. Indirectly, pepsin activity which is necessary for digestion can be decreased by increasing the pH of gastric juice from 1 or 2 to a pH of 4 or 5. Total neutralization (pH 7.0) inactivates pepsin activity. Some antacids (those with aluminum, calcium or bismuth) inhibit pepsin activity directly.

a. **NON-SYSTEMIC ANTACIDS**: These compounds have a cationic group which can form insoluble basic compounds that are not absorbed but are excreted to avoid production of alkalosis.

CALCIUM SALTS:

Calcium Carbonate: Rapid neutralization can cause belching (CO_2 gas forms). Unpleasant chalky taste, precipitates in GI tract to cause constipation. Hypercalcemia can occur with chronic usage if large amounts of milk and dairy products ingested - "milk-alkali syndrome".

MAGNESIUM SALTS

Magnesium Hydroxide: (Milk of Magnesia) An antacid as well as a laxative. Has a laxative effect which is lessened by use with $CaCO_3$ or $Al(OH)_3$, which tend to produce constipation. Some absorption and retention of magnesium (if renal function impaired) could produce neurological or cardiovascular toxicity.
Magnesium Trisilicate: Reacts with acid to form Si_3O_2; has gelatinous form; thought to adhere to the ulcer and to form a protective coating (a demulcent effect); slow onset of action; diarrhea may be produced.

ALUMINUM SALTS

Aluminum Hydroxide: Remains in stomach for long periods and slowly reacts with stomach acid to form aluminum chloride. It may inhibit action of pepsin and stimulate stomach mucus secretion. Aluminum compounds produce constipation. They can interfere with phosphate absorption to cause osteomalacia and also can decrease absorption of the tetracyclines, other antibiotics and drugs.
Basic Aluminum Carbonate: Similar to $Al(OH)_3$; recommended for phosphatic nephrolithiasis; binds more phosphate than other aluminum-containing antacids.
Aluminum Phosphate: Will not reduce phosphate levels and is used in patients where this problem should be avoided.

ANTACID MIXTURES: Because of the constipating effects of aluminum or calcium salts and the laxative effects of magnesium salts, these salts are combined in over-the-counter and prescription preparations to avoid these unwanted effects.

b. **SYSTEMIC ANTACIDS**: Have a cationic group that is not capable of forming insoluble basic compounds; such agents may produce metabolic alkalosis.

Sodium bicarbonate: Highly soluble; rapidly neutralizes acid; produces lots of CO_2 causing episodes of burping; severe distention of stomach with by CO_2 gas may be dangerous if a gastric ulcer is present that could perforate; contraindicated in edema and heart failure.

4. Sucralfate: Thought to accelerate healing of duodenal ulcers by forming a protective barrier over ulcer base; forms an ulcer-adherent complex with proteinaceous exudate at the ulcer site; not absorbed; does not inhibit acid secretion or neutralize acid; thought to protect ulcer from pepsin; minimal adverse reactions, constipation; may bind digoxin or tetracyclines.

5. Misoprostol: A prostaglandin derivative that has both cytoprotective and anti-secretory actions. Given orally, it can cause diarrhea and some abdominal cramping.

6. Metoclopramide: Dopamine antagonist. A prokinetic agent that stimulates gastric emptying and increases esophageal sphincter tone, thus is useful in reflex esophagitis. Its antiemetic effects also make it useful in treating the nausea associated with cancer chemotherapy.

7. Pirenzepine: This is a tricyclic anticholinergic drug apparently with selective activity to inhibit M_1 subtype muscarinic receptors on the parietal cells of the stomach.

8. Anticholinergics: General anticholinergics are not very useful because they are non-selective and the large doses required to inhibit gastric acid secretion produced by parasympathetic nerve activity cause too many unpleasant side effects.

B. ESOPHAGEAL DISORDERS

Metoclopramide: Dopamine antagonist which is useful in reflux esophagitis.
Histamine H_2 blockers may relieve pain but do not affect sphincter tone.

C. DIGESTANTS

Agents used in deficiency conditions to promote the digestion of food by the GI
tract.
Pepsin: Proteolytic enzyme; sometimes used with HCl to treat gastric achylia, in
people suffering from pernicious anemia or stomach cancer.
HCl: Dilute solutions of HCl for gastric hypochlorhydria or achlorhydria;
encountered in pernicious anemia, stomach cancer, gastritis and in the elderly.
Pancreatic Enzymes: Available as pancreatin, a powder from hog pancreas,
containing enzymes trypsin, steapsin and amylopsin. Used where there is deficient
secretion of pancreatic juice, such as pancreatitis.

D. DRUGS TO DISSOLVE GALLSTONES

Chenodiol: A primary bile acid which is used to dissolve cholesterol gallstones;
dose-related diarrhea frequent; limited usefulness.

E. EMETICS

Therapeutic interventions in treating poisonings may involve measures to
remove unabsorbed substances and/or the prevention of absorption of remaining
substance.
Ipecac Syrup: Stimulates the chemoreceptor trigger zone (CTZ); also irritates the
GI tract; must give within 4 hrs after ingesting a poison, emesis occurs within 5-20
min; contraindicated in coma, convulsions, and after ingestion of caustic (corrosive)
agents; also caution with petroleum hydrocarbons, may get severe aspiration
pneumonitis.
Apomorphine: Derived by treating morphine with a strong mineral acid; stimulates
the CTZ; also a dopaminergic agonist; s.c. administration usually produces emesis
within 5 min.; clinical usefulness is limited because it can cause CNS and
respiratory depression.

F. ANTI-EMETIC DRUGS

<u>Stimulus for emesis:</u>

1. Irritation of sensory G.I. nerve endings ($CuSO_4$)
2. Agents acting on CTZ (chemoreceptor trigger zone in medulla (apomorphine, morphine, digitalis, i.v. $CuSO_4$)
3. Emotional or psychic vomiting
4. Motion sickness

5. Nausea and vomiting of pregnancy

6. Nausea and vomiting of cancer chemotherapy

<u>Blocked by:</u>

1. Vagotomy
2. Blocked competitively by phenothiazines

3. Blocked by sedative-hypnotics
4. Blocked by drugs having <u>CNS anticholinergic</u> action
   a) Scopolamine and benztropine
   b) Antihistamines with CNS anticholinergic actions diphenhydramine, cyclizine, and dimenhydrinate
   c) <u>Promethazine</u> - a phenothiazine with CNS anticholinergic effects
5. Because of concerns about teratogenicity, drugs should not be used unless absolutely necessary. If vomiting persists, may consider cyclizine, meclizine and promethazine
6. Phenothiazines (prochlorperazine), cannabinoids (nabilone), metoclopramide and drug combinations

II. LOWER GI DISORDERS

A. LAXATIVES AND CATHARTICS

These terms describe drugs that promote defecation; a laxative promotes excretion of a soft formed stool; a cathartic promotes a more fluid evacuation.

1. CONTACT (STIMULANT-IRRITANT) CATHARTICS

Increase intestinal motor activity and stimulate water and electrolyte accumulation in the colon.

Castor Oil: Oil from the seeds of Ricinus Communis; pancreatic lipases hydrolyze the oil to the active irritant agent, ricinoleic acid; acts on the small intestine in 1-3 hrs; should not be used just prior to bedtime; disagreeable taste.

Diphenylmethanes: Phenolphthalein and bisacodyl act in 6-8 hrs. given at bedtime to produce effect the following morning. Phenolphthalein is a widely used proprietary cathartic in gums and candy; if alkaline, the excreted phenolphthalein will turn the urine and feces red; allergic reactions may occur.

Anthraquinones: Active ingredient of Cascara, senna and Danthron is anthraquinone or its derivatives; act on the large intestine in 6 to 8 hrs.

2. BULK-FORMING LAXATIVES

Naturally-occurring or synthetic polysaccharides; absorb and retain water; fecal material becomes hydrated and soft; may also act to reflexly stimulate peristalsis; act within 1-3 days; intestinal obstruction reported; some drug absorption may be reduced by binding to these agents.

Bran and other dietary fiber
Methylcellulose and sodium carboxymethylcellulose
Psyllium preparations

3. SALINE (OSMOTIC) CATHARTICS

This group includes sulfates, phosphates, tartrates and magnesium salts; they are poorly and slowly absorbed from the GI tract. Water is retained by an osmotic effect to indirectly increase peristalsis; watery evacuation occurs in less than 3 hours; approximately 20% of Mg^{++} absorbed but it is rapidly excreted if renal function is normal; Mg^{++} intoxication can occur if renal function impaired.

Magnesium sulfate   Magnesium Citrate
Milk of Magnesia   Potassium or Sodium Phosphate

4. EMOLLIENT LAXATIVES (Fecal Softeners)

No direct or reflex stimulation of peristalsis occurs with these agents; use is limited; feces kept soft and tenesmus (straining at stool) is avoided.

Surface Active Agents: Dioctyl sodium (or calcium) sulfosuccinate produces softening within 1-2 days; lowers surface tension to promote water penetration into feces.

5. **LUBRICANT LAXATIVES**

<u>Mineral Oil</u>: A mixture of liquid hydrocarbons obtained from petroleum; retards reabsorption of water; use discouraged because of adverse effects; can produce lipid pneumonia in elderly or debilitated patients; foreign-body reactions in mesenteric lymph nodes, liver, spleen and intestinal mucosa; absorption of essential fat soluble substances (vitamin A, carotene, and vitamins K and D) may be blocked.

6. **VALID USES OF CATHARTICS AND LAXATIVES**

Include radiological exams of GI tract; bowel surgery; proctological exam; for patients with a hernia or cardiovascular disease or in anorectal disorders (such as hemorrhoids), after anthelminthic therapy or poisoning by drugs or foods. These agents are contraindicated in the presence of colic, nausea, vomiting, cramps, undiagnosed abdominal pain, and symptoms of appendicitis

7. **SPECIALIZED LAXATIVE FOR CHRONIC LIVER DISEASE**

<u>Lactulose</u>: Used in hepatic coma to decrease plasma levels of ammonia. Given orally but not absorbed. Intestinal bacteria hydrolyze the drug which leads to a more acid pH of colon. This reduces ability of bacteria to form ammonia.

B. **ANTI-DIARRHEAL AGENTS**

1. **ADSORBENTS**

Supposedly inert powders have been employed for the treatment of diarrhea and dysentery. Severe diarrhea quickly can cause serious dehydration and electrolyte imbalance. Nonspecific therapy may prolong the course of an enteric infection.
<u>Bismuth Subcarbonate</u>: Heavy, white powder; given in aqueous suspension.
<u>Kaolin</u>: Hydrated aluminum silicate; often given in a mixture with pectin.
<u>Pectin</u>: A purified carbohydrate from acid extracts of apples or the rinds of citrus fruits.
   Reduce tone and motility of GI tract; common side effects, dryness of the mouth, photophobia, blurred vision and tachycardia.

2. **OPIOIDS**

   These agents decrease propulsion and peristalsis; G.I. contents are delayed in passage allowing time for feces to become desiccated; this further retards passage through the colon. Effective in acute diarrheal states but should not use for enteric infections.

Opium Alkaloids: Effective for controlling severe diarrhea or dysentery; with chronic therapy there is a risk of dependence.

Paregoric: Camphorated tincture of opium; an agent which was widely used for centuries, especially for infantile diarrhea,

Codeine and/or morphine: Purified opium alkaloids which are very poorly absorbed after oral administration. They exert a local action in the gastrointestinal tract.

Diphenoxylate: A congener of meperidine; high or chronic doses lead to euphoria and physical dependence; often given in combination with atropine.

Difenoxan + atropine: The principle active metabolite of diphenoxylate.

Loperamide: A derivative of haloperidol that resembles meperidine. Appears to be as effective as diphenoxylate with few side effects reported. This drug is often used for the prophylaxis and treatment of travelers' diarrhea.

REVIEW QUESTIONS

ONE BEST ANSWER

1. Which cathartics or laxatives should not be taken just before going to bed?

   A. Cascara
   B. Danthron
   C. Methylcellulose
   D. Phenolphthalein
   E. Castor oil

2. Which of the following cathartics or laxatives is a bulk-forming agent?

   A. Castor oil
   B. Danthron
   C. Milk of magnesia
   D. Methyl or carboxymethylcellulose
   E. Phenolphthalein

3. Side effects including pneumonia in the elderly, foreign-body reactions, and interference with the absorption of fat-soluble vitamins are most likely to be seen with:

   A. Mineral oil
   B. Danthron
   C. Phenolphthalein
   D. Epsom salts
   E. Milk of magnesia

4. Each of the following statements about antacids is true **EXCEPT**:

   A. They are used for treatment of peptic ulcer
   B. They are used for treatment of hyperchlorhydria
   C. They are weak bases
   D. They decrease pepsin activity by decreasing the stomach pH to 1
   E. Those containing Al or Cl also have a direct effect to inhibit pepsin activity

5. Unpleasant side effects of anticholinergics when used to inhibit acid secretion in patients with peptic ulcers include all of the following **EXCEPT**:

   A. Dryness of the mouth
   B. Increased tone of the GI tract
   C. Photophobia
   D. Blurred vision
   E. Tachycardia

6. Which of the following is the most effective agent for treatment of severe diarrhea or dysentery?

   A. Opium alkaloid
   B. Kaolin
   C. Pectin
   D. Bismuth subcarbonate
   E. Gamma globulin

7. Which of the following induces emesis by a direct action on the medullary chemoreceptor trigger zone (CTZ)?

   A. Apomorphine
   B. Hydroxyzine
   C. Nabilone
   D. Chlorpromazine
   E. Diphenhydramine

8. Which of the following is likely to cause systemic alkalosis when used orally as an antacid?

   A. Sodium bicarbonate
   B. Calcium carbonate
   C. Aluminum hydroxide
   D. Magnesium hydroxide
   E. Basic aluminum carbonate

9. Diphenoxylate:

   A. Is an opioid-like drug
   B. Is an atropine-like anticholinergic
   C. Is an irritant cathartic
   D. is an antiemetic agent
   E. Is an antisecretory agent

MATCHING

   A. Omeprazole
   B. Pirenzepine
   C. Metoclopramide
   D. Cimetidine
   E. Misoprostol

10. Blocks M_1 receptors on gastric parietal cell

11. Proton pump inhibitor

12. Has both cytoprotective and antisecretory actions

CHAPTER 13: RESPIRATORY DRUGS

I. DRUGS USED FOR ASTHMA

ASTHMA: Asthma is predominantly an inflammatory disease with associated bronchospasm. It is characterized by bronchial hyperreactivity with episodic bronchial obstruction that can be manifested by wheezing, dyspnea, cough and mucosal edema. Children may have only a persistent cough.

A. Treatment of acute asthma or status asthmaticus

    1. Oxygen and i.v. fluids for hydration to thin mucous secretions
    2. ß-Adrenergic agonists
       a. albuterol or metaproterenol by nebulizer
       b. terbutaline or epinephrine by s.c. injection
    3. Intravenous glucocorticoids if ß-adrenergic agonists do not provide improvement
    4. Theophylline by i.v. infusion; usefulness has been questioned by some authorities

B. Treatment and management of chronic asthma

    1. <u>Mild asthma</u>: An inhaled ß$_2$ adrenergic agonist (albuterol, terbutaline or metaproterenol) should be used prior to exposure to factors that provoke asthma or at the first manifestation of symptoms.
    2. <u>Moderate asthma</u>: Inhaled glucocorticoids, cromolyn sodium or other antiinflammatory agents are recommended for the initial treatment. Prolonged-release oral theophylline and a long-acting ß$_2$ adrenergic agonist, either alone or in combination, are the main therapies.
    3. <u>Severe asthma</u>: Oral glucocorticoids are given to prevent acute episodes.

C. Drugs used in asthma therapy

    1. *Adrenal corticosteroids*: These antiinflammatory agents are the most effective antiasthmatic drugs available. In addition to inflammation, they decrease bronchial hyperreactivity and the formation of mucus.
       a. Oral <u>prednisone</u> or <u>methylprednisone</u> can be taken daily for up to two weeks. When longer periods of therapy are necessary, these agents should be given on alternate days to avoid adrenal suppression.
       b. <u>Beclomethasone</u> or <u>triamcinolone</u> are given by inhalation and they can be used prophylactically after control of severe asthma with oral glucocorticoids is achieved.   Adverse effects, such as throat irritation and dysphonia, may limit compliance. Fungal infections are possible with improper technique of administration. The potential for adrenal suppression must be considered when changing from oral preparations to inhaled preparations.

2. <u>Cromolyn sodium</u>: This agents blocks various inflammation cascade reactions and reduces bronchial hyperresponsiveness. Cromolyn may be used for initial therapy in mild asthma, particularly for prophylaxis in children. It is used for allergic, seasonal or occupational asthma and for or exercise-induced asthma; side effects are minimal..

3. *Adrenergic bronchodilators*: <u>Albuterol</u>, <u>terbutaline</u> and <u>metaproterenol</u> are selective agonists for β_2-adrenoceptors. They can rapidly reverse bronchoconstriction and provide symptomatic relief but they do not decrease significantly the bronchial hyperresponsiveness or the primary inflammatory reactions responsible for the persistence of asthma. Tremor, anxiety and restlessness are the most common adverse effects.

4. *Methylxanthines*: <u>Theophylline</u> and <u>aminophylline</u> are still the most prescribed bronchodilators for maintenance therapy of moderate to severe asthma. Prolonged-release oral or intravenous formulations are most commonly used. Monitoring of serum levels is essential because of large interindividual variability. Life-threatening toxicity (seizures and cardiac arrhythmias) can occur at high doses without warning signs. Nausea, cramps, insomnia and headache are common with loading doses.

5. *Anticholinergic drugs*: <u>Ipratropium</u> or atropine have limited efficacy in asthma. They may be useful by reducing a high level of cholinergic tone that may contribute to reflex bronchoconstriction.

II. OTHER RESPIRATORY DISORDERS

A. CHRONIC OBSTRUCTIVE AIRWAY DISEASE (COAD): Chronic obstructive bronchitis, emphysema and asthma can coexist. Oxygen and antibiotic therapy are important. <u>Ipratropium</u> is the drug of choice for bronchodilation of a syndrome with a reversible airway blockage. α_1 <u>Proteinase inhibitor</u> is indicated for patients with panacinar emphysema who have α_1 antitrypsin deficiency.

B. NEONATAL RESPIRATORY DISTRESS SYNDROME: Hyaline membrane disease is caused by a deficiency in surfactant. This syndrome can be modulated by administering the agent, <u>beractant</u>, a modified bovine lung extract (a natural surfactant) and <u>colfosceril</u> (a synthetic surfactant). These agents are given by tracheal instillation.

C. RHINITIS: <u>Antihistamines</u> are commonly used for allergic rhinitis. They are effective prophylactically in relieving rhinorrhea, sneezing and conjunctivitis but do not counteract nasal congestion. <u>α-Adrenergic agonists</u> are used for nasal decongestion. The corticosteroid, <u>dexamethasone</u>, is the most effective agent available for prophylaxis and treatment of allergic rhinitis. It is administered as a nasal spray and its use should be limited to 30 days of treatment. These agents are not effective for the common cold.

REVIEW QUESTIONS

ONE BEST ANSWER

1. The reason that the effective therapeutic concentration of theophylline is lower in infants than that measured in adults is because of:

   A. Decreased absorption
   B. Slower metabolism
   C. Decreased protein binding
   D. Increased receptor sensitivity
   E. Increased receptor density

2. The only therapeutic agent for chronic obstructive airway disease that has been shown conclusively to enhance survival is:
   A. Methylprednisolone
   B. Tetracycline
   C. Theophylline
   D. Oxygen
   E. Cromolyn

3. In emphysema patients with inadequate elastase activity, the drug of choice is which one of the following?

   A. Ipratropium
   B. α_1 proteinase inhibitor
   C. Beractant
   D. Pancrelipase
   E. Rifampin

4. Which one of the following is the most effective antiasthmatic drug?

   A. Albuterol
   B. Theophylline
   C. Cromolyn sodium
   D. Beclomethasone
   E. Prednisone

MATCHING: Use a letter only once.

   A. Cromolyn
   B. Theophylline
   C. Beclomethasone
   D. Ipratropium
   E. Albuterol

5. Drug of choice for chronic obstructive airway disease

6. Methylxanthine used in asthma

7. Selective β_2-adrenoceptor agonist

8. Stabilizes mast cells

9. Potential for adrenal suppression

CHAPTER 14: <u>DRUGS ACTING ON THE UTERUS</u>

I. **OXYTOCIC DRUGS**

    A. **OXYTOCIN (See Posterior Pituitary Hormones, Endocrine Section for general information).**

       1. PROPERTIES:

         a. Oxytocin is one of 2 fractions extracted from the posterior pituitary gland; it is now prepared synthetically .

         b. The uterus is more sensitive to vasopressin than oxytocin except in the third trimester of pregnancy.

         c. During the third trimester, uterine oxytocin receptors increase in number, and sensitivity to oxytocin is maximal at term (vasopressin sensitivity decreases in parallel). Estrogen has a "priming effect" on the uterus.

         d. Oxytocin causes myoepithelial cells of the mammary gland to contract, and stimulates milk "let-down".

         e. Oxytocin causes a transient fall in blood pressure when injected i.v.

         f. Oxytocin is ineffective orally (destroyed by stomach enzymes) and is usually given i.v. or i.m.. It is also absorbed through oral or nasal mucosa.

         g. Uterine contractions occur within seconds after i.v. injection and last about 20 minutes.

       2. CLINICAL USES:

         a. Induce labor at term

         b. Promote milk ejection in cases of inadequacy of breast feeding

         c. Relief of breast engorgement during lactation

         d. Control post-partum hemorrhage

       3. ADVERSE REACTIONS:

         a. Sodium and water retention

         b. Do not use in patients with uterine abnormalities

       4. PREPARATIONS:

         a. Oxytocin injection

         b. Nasal spray

B. PROSTAGLANDINS

1. PROPERTIES:

    a. Prostaglandins have a long duration of action, and may produce a wide variety of unpleasant side effects.
    b. Prostaglandins can stimulate the pregnant and non-pregnant uterus.
    c. In the first trimester of pregnancy, prostaglandins have a low success rate inducing abortion.
    d. PGE_1 PGE_2 or $PGF_{2\alpha}$ could be used to induce labor at term. However, oxytocin is used because its short duration of action allows better control over progression of labor.

2. PREPARATIONS:

    a. Carboprost tromethamine (synthetic analog of $PGF_{2\alpha}$)
    b. Dinoprostone (PGE_2)

C. ERGOT ALKALOIDS

Ergot (Claviceps purpurea) is a fungus which grows on rye. Extracts of ergot contain a variety of pharmacologically active substances (histamine, tyramine, etc.). Ergot alkaloids per se are derivatives of lysergic acid. Chronic ergot poisoning is associated with gangrene of extremities caused by severe vasoconstriction, convulsive (CNS) effects and spontaneous abortion. Ergot alkaloids have varied actions as agonists or antagonists on tryptaminergic, dopaminergic and adrenergic receptors.

1. ERGONOVINE:

    a. Most potent ergot compound for oxytocic effect; relatively selective action on the uterus.
    b. Can cause forceful, prolonged or sustained contractions.
    c. Rapid absorption after oral administration provides prompt onset of action.
    d. Partial α-adrenergic receptor agonist.
    e. Chief uses - to prevent and treat postpartum hemorrhage (after delivery of the placenta); to hasten involution of the uterus.

2. METHYLERGONOVINE: A semisynthetic derivative with similar properties as ergonovine

II. **UTERINE RELAXANTS (Tocolytic Drugs)**

A. **INDICATIONS**

1. To delay or prevent premature birth.
2. To slow labor in order to prepare for complicated delivery.

B. **ß$_2$ ADRENERGIC AGONISTS**

RITODRINE has been approved for tocolytic use. Its adverse effects are typical of all β_2 agonists, and include increased cardiac output, hydration, hyperglycemia, and hypokalemia. Terbutaline is an alternative drug.

C. **MAGNESIUM SULFATE**

Given i.v., stops contractions at Mg^{++} concentrations of 4-8 mg/dl through direct inhibition of action potentials in myometrial muscle cells. Magnesium sulfate is used to control convulsions in patients with eclampsia and pre-eclampsia.

207

REVIEW QUESTIONS

ONE BEST ANSWER

1. Emesis associated with injection of ergot derivatives is relatively minimal with:

    A. Methysergide
    B. Methylergonovine
    C. Ergonovine
    D. Ergotamine
    E. Dihydroergotamine

2. Both the absorption and peripheral actions of ergotamine are enhanced by:

    A. Sumatripan
    B. Epinephrine
    C. Caffeine
    D. Propranolol
    E. Alcohol

3. Retroperitoneal fibrosis is a possible complication of long-term therapy with:

    A. Methylprednisolone
    B. Penicillamine
    C. Dimercaprol
    D. Methysergide
    E. Sumatripan

4. Limits are placed on the amount of this drug that can be taken per week, because of the risk of drug accumulation and associated vasoconstriction:

    A. EDTA
    B. Dimercaprol
    C. Sumatripan
    D. Vasopressin
    E. Ergotamine

MATCHING: Use a letter only once

    A. Methylergonovine
    B. Magnesium sulfate
    C. Carboprost tromethamine
    D. Oxytocin
    E. Ritodrine

5. Given intravenously to control convulsions in eclampsia

6. Used as a nasal spray for relief of breast engorgement

7. Orally effective tocolytic agent

8. Used for second trimester abortions

9. Orally effective to control post partum bleeding

CHAPTER 15: <u>TOXICOLOGY</u>

I. **EMERGENCY TREATMENT OF THE POISONED PATIENT**

First check respiratory function, cardiovascular function, CNS involvement, and stabilize the patient. Then attempt to determine the identity and quantity of poison ingested, and the time of exposure.

A. NON-SPECIFIC ANTIDOTES:

1. Emetics:
   a. <u>Syrup of ipecac</u>: One ounce orally usually produces emesis within 30 min.
   b. <u>Apomorphine</u>: Given by injection, produces emesis in 1-3 minutes
2. <u>Activated charcoal</u>: Adsorbs a large number of organic and inorganic compounds and prevents their absorption from the GI tract. Given orally as a suspension in doses of up to 100 grams.
3. Saline cathartics: Reduce contact time between the poison and absorption sites. Examples - magnesium or sodium sulfate, magnesium citrate.
4. Diuretics: Forced diuresis may help to eliminate compounds excreted into urine. Agents used include mannitol and furosemide.

   Urinary excretion may further be enhanced by acidification or alkalinization of the urine. Weak bases (e.g. amphetamine, phencyclidine) are excreted faster ("ion-trapped") if the urine is acidified with ascorbic acid or ammonium chloride. Acidic drugs (e.g. salicylates) will be excreted faster if the urine is alkalinized with sodium bicarbonate.

B. SPECIFIC ANTIDOTES:

When the identity of the toxic substances is known or strongly suspected, it may be desirable to treat with specific antidotes.

Examples of Specific Antidotes

Poison	Antidote and Comments
Belladonna (Atropine)	Physostigmine - anticholinesterase action
Carbon monoxide	Hyperbaric O_2 - increases both O_2 delivery to tissue and CO elimination
Coumarin Derivatives	Phytonadione (Vitamin K_1)
Cyanide	Sodium thiosulfate - increases cyanide metabolism Amyl nitrite, sodium nitrite - produce methemoglobin which binds cyanide
Ethylene glycol, and other glycols	Ethanol - preferentially metabolized by alcohol dehydrogenase, prevents occurrence of acidosis
Iodine	Starch - binds iodine
Methanol	Ethanol - preferentially metabolized by alcohol dehydrogenase and decreases formation of formaldehyde and formic acid from methanol
Narcotics	Naloxone - narcotic antagonist
Nitrites	Methylene blue - reduces methemoglobin to hemoglobin
Organophosphate Insecticides	Pralidoxime - cholinesterase reactivator Atropine - anticholinergic agent

II. HEAVY METALS

A. LEAD:

1. Acute intoxication is rare. Symptoms of chronic intoxications include:
   a. GI: intestinal smooth muscle stimulated; spasm and hypermotility cause intense cramping - lead colic
   b. CNS: lead encephalopathy - primarily a problem in children; early symptoms rather non-specific; decreased appetite, irritability, fatigue abdominal pain, vomiting - followed by drowsiness, stupor convulsions, and coma. May lead to mental retardation in survivors; may also cause cerebral palsies.

     c. Neuromuscular: lead palsy - myopathy; fatigue, weakness; wrist drop; foot drop; involvement of extra-ocular muscles;

     d. Also see anemia due to impaired heme biosynthesis; porphyrinuria, basophilic stippling of erythrocytes; gingival lead line. Blood vessel constriction causes pallor and hypertension.

     e. Treatment: Edetate for initial treatment; penicillamine also has been used; effectiveness of dimercaprol is limited.

B. MERCURY:

1. Acute: greatest danger is damage of GI mucosa and kidney; fluid loss leads to shock and death.
2. Chronic: characterized by stomatitis, excessive salivation and blue gumline; renal toxicity; CNS symptoms (depression, weakness, headache, insomnia, irritability, hallucinations).
3. Treatment: Dimercaprol

C. IRON:

1. Most common metallic poison, due to overdosage with oral supplements, multiple transfusions, or iron storage diseases.

III. METAL CHELATING AGENTS

A. DIMERCAPROL (British Anti-Lewisite, BAL):

1. Effective for poisoning by mercury, arsenic and some other less common metals; not very effective for lead poisoning; given i.m.
2. Protects essential enzymes by forming stable complex with circulating metallic poison; promotes excretion of metal in stable complex form.
3. Adverse effects: increased blood pressure and heart rate; weakness, nausea, pain at injection site.

B. CALCIUM DISODIUM EDETATE (CaNa$_2$EDTA):

1. Especially effective in lead poisoning; given by i.v. drip; may be useful to chelate other less common metallic poisons; not effective orally.
2. Promotes excretion of the lead chelate.
3. Adverse effects: renal damage, hypersensitivity reactions

C. PENICILLAMINE:

1. Chelates copper, mercury, lead; given orally.
2. Used to remove copper in hepatolenticular degeneration (Wilson's disease) - accumulation of copper in tissues.
3. Used in combination, usually after EDTA for lead poisoning.

4. Adverse effects: hypersensitivity reactions; rashes arthralgia, nephrotic syndrome. TRIENTINE is an alternative copper chelating agent for hypersensitive patients.

D. DEFEROXAMINE:

1. Chelates iron specifically; orally effective to prevent iron absorption; given i.m. or i.v. for systemic toxicity.
2. Used for acute iron toxicity, iron storage diseases.
3. Adverse effects: increased blood pressure, rashes, GI upset.

E. SUCCIMER:

1. Orally effective drug indicated for lead poisoning in children.
2. May also be effective for mercury or arsenic.

IV. TERATOGENESIS

A. Most teratogenic effects of drugs occur during the first trimester of pregnancy.

B. Teratogenic effects may be species-specific, which complicates drug toxicity testing.

C. In some cases, adverse complications of a disease state (e.g. epilepsy) may pose more risk to the developing fetus than drugs used to control the symptoms.

V. CHEMICAL CARCINOGENESIS

Many chemicals which are present as industrial or environmental pollutants, dietary components, combustion by-products or therapeutic agents may increase the risk of cancer development. Two main classifications of chemical carcinogens have been proposed, based on their apparent mechanisms of action.

A. GENOTOXIC CARCINOGENS:

Most chemical carcinogens are thought to initiate tumorigenesis by interacting with DNA. Chemicals may be inherently genotoxic, but many chemical carcinogens are metabolized to highly reactive metabolites which in turn damage DNA. Alternatively, chemicals could act by altering DNA replication or repair.

B. EPIGENETIC CARCINOGENS:

Epigenetic carcinogens do not appear to interact directly with DNA, but appear to augment neoplastic growth by poorly defined mechanisms. This class of carcinogens includes various hormones (e.g. estrogen, diethylstilbestrol), immunosuppressive drugs (e.g. azathioprine), solid-state carcinogens (e.g. asbestos), and promoting agents (agents which increase tumor development when given after a genotoxic chemical).

REVIEW QUESTIONS

ONE BEST ANSWER

1. An oily metal chelating agent with a disagreeable odor, which is given by i.m. injection:

   A. Dimercaprol
   B. Calcium disodium edetate
   C. Penicillamine
   D. Succimer
   E. Deferoxamine

2. If patients with Wilson's Disease become allergic to penicillamine, an alternative drug is:

   A. EDTA
   B. Dimercaprol
   C. Succimer
   D. Trientine
   E. Magnesium citrate

3. Teratogenic effects of drugs:

   A. Are easily predicted from animal studies
   B. Result in an absolute contraindication of their use during any stage of pregnancy
   C. Are most likely to occur during the first trimester
   D. Are most likely to occur in the second trimester
   E. Are most likely to occur in the third trimester

4. Irritability, hallucinations, and blue gumline are symptoms of chronic poisoning with:

   A. Lead
   B. Arsenic
   C. Mercury
   D. Iron
   E. Cadmium

5. A patient who has received multiple blood transfusions may require chelation therapy with:

   A. Dimercaprol
   B. Succimer
   C. EDTA
   D. Trientine
   E. Deferoxamine

MATCHING: Use a letter only once

Match the antidote from the following list with its indication:

A. Activated charcoal
B. Apomorphine
C. Dimercaprol
D. Edetate
E. Ethanol
F. Flumazenil
G. Ipecac syrup
H. Nitrites, amyl or sodium
I. Penicillamine
J. Physostigmine
K. Phytonadione
L. Pralidoxime
M. Specific antibody fragments
N. Succimer

6. Orally effective copper chelating agent

7. Antidote for ethylene glycol ingestion

8. Benzodiazepine antagonist

9. Emetic effects are blocked by naloxone

10. Orally effective chelating agent for lead poisoning in children

11. Specific antidote for ingestion of warfarin-based rodenticides

12. Administered along with thiosulfate in cyanide poisoning

13. Antagonist for belladonna alkaloids

14. The oral dose in treatment of acute oral poisoning may be as high as 50 grams

15. Orally effective emetic agent

16. Used in cases of digoxin overdose

17. Administered along with atropine in treatment of parathion poisoning

CHAPTER 16: <u>WATER-SOLUBLE VITAMINS</u>

Vitamin	Biochemical Function	Deficiency	Therapeutic Use	Toxicity
Thiamine (B$_1$)	Essential for carbo-hydrate metabolism; modulator of neurotransmitter activity	Beriberi: neurological (dry) or cardiovascular (wet)	Deficiency state	None recognized
Riboflavin (B$_2$)	In FMN and FAD, functions in hydrogen transport	Cheilosis, angular stomatitis, glossitis, seborrheic dermatitis of nose & scrotum, ocular symptoms	Deficiency state	None recognized
Niacin (nicotinic acid)	In NAD(P)(H), cofactors for numerous dehydrogenases	Pellagra, "three D's: dermatitis, diarrhea, dementia	Deficiency due to malabsorption, alcoholism, isoniazid therapy; Hartnup disease, carcinoid; elevated blood lipids	Flushing, headache, pruritus, GI irritation
Pyridoxine (B$_6$)	Functions in amino acid and protein metabolism	Seizures, anemia, homocystinuria, cystathioninuria	Vitamin B complex deficiency; deficiency due to inborn errors of metabolism, therapy with isoniazid, cycloserine, hydralazine	Sensory neuropathy, interference with levodopa therapy
Pantothenic Acid	Precursor for CoA	Spontaneous clinical deficiency has not been observed	Multivitamin therapy	None recognized

WATER-SOLUBLE VITAMINS

Vitamin	Biochemical Function	Deficiency	Therapeutic Use	Toxicity
Biotin	Coenzyme essential for fatty acid and carbohydrate metabolism	Alopecia, anorexia, mental depression, memory loss, dermatitis	Deficiency due to inborn error of metabolism; multiple carboxylase deficiency	None recognized
Folic acid	Cofactor in 1-carbon transfer reactions	Megaloblastic anemia	Deficiency state	None recognized
Vitamin B_{12} (Cyano-cobalamine)	Component of various coenzymes, important in synthesis of nucleic acid and of myelin	Megaloblastic anemia, neurologic symptoms	Deficiency state	None recognized
Ascorbic Acid (vitamin C)	Cofactor in hydroxylation and amidation reactions, provides reducing equivalents; important for collagen biosynthesis, neurotransmitter synthesis, intestinal absorption of iron	Scurvy: hemorrhages, loose teeth, gingivitis, anemia	Prevention or treatment of scurvy	With megadoses: kidney stones, rebound scurvy

FAT-SOLUBLE VITAMINS

Vitamin	Biochemical Function	Deficiency	Therapeutic Use	Toxicity
Vitamin A (retinol)	Important for growth, bone development, integrity of mucosal and epithelial surfaces, vision, reproduction	Night blindness, hyperkeratosis of skin, metaplasia of mucosa	Deficiency states, prophylaxis, acne, other skin diseases	Acute: dizziness, vomiting, erythema, desquamation Chronic: skin & hair changes, liver damage; in infants & children pseudomotor cerebri, increased CSF pressure
Vitamin D (ergocalciferol, D₂; chole-calciferol, D₂)	Regulates calcium homeostasis	Decreased bone density, rickets, osteomalacia	Deficiency states, prophylaxis, hypoparathyroidism	Hypercalcemia, mental and physical retardation
Vitamin E (tocopherol)	Antioxidant; important for vitamin A utilization, neuronal maintenance	In experimental animals, adverse effects on nervous, reproductive, muscular, cardiovascular, & hematopoietic systems	Retinopathy of prematurity, vitamin E deficiency due to malabsorption	Nausea, muscular weakness, fatigue, headache, blurred vision, GI upset
Vitamin K (phytonadione, menadione)	Promotes hepatic synthesis of factors II, VII, IX and X	Hypoprothrombinemia, tendency to bleed	Vitamin K deficiency due to malabsorption, cleansing of the bowel, antibiotic or anticoagulant therapy,	Hemolytic anemia, hyperbilirubinemia in newborns & G6PD people

REVIEW QUESTIONS

MATCHING: Use a letter only once.

Match the appropriate vitamins with their therapeutic indications.

    A. Folic acid
    B. Vitamin E
    C. Ascorbic acid
    D. Niacin
    E. Vitamin D

1. Prevention of scurvy.

2. Hartnup disease

3. Retinopathy of prematurity

4. Prevention of rickets

5. Megaloblastic anemia

MATCHING: Use a letter only once.

Match the vitamins with their associated toxicities.

    A. Niacin
    B. Pyridoxine (B_6)
    C. Vitamin K (phytonadione)
    D. Vitamin D (ergocalciferol D_2)
    E. Vitamin A (retinol)

6. Hypercalcemia

7. Sensory neuropathy

8. Chronic skin and hair changes; liver damage

9. Hemolytic anemia

10. Flushing, headache

CHAPTER 17: <u>U.S. DRUG LAWS</u>

THE FOOD, DRUG, AND COSMETIC ACT of 1938 and amendments to this law govern all aspects of drug development, testing, marketing and distribution in the United States. The FOOD AND DRUG ADMINISTRATION has the responsibility of enforcement of the drug laws, testing products to assure that they meet established standards of quality, assuring drug safety and efficacy, etc.

I. NEW DRUG DEVELOPMENT

When a pharmaceutical firm wishes to market a new drug in the United States, testing for chemical stability and safety in animals is required before the FDA will approve an IND (Investigational New Drug) application. Under an approved IND, phase I, II, and III clinical trials are conducted. If the drug continues to show promise, an NDA (New Drug Application) is filed with the FDA. The FDA may approve the marketing of the drug only after careful review of all data accumulated during the development of the drug.

II. DRUG SAFETY

Several large-scale examples of drug toxicity (e.g., thalidomide, sulfanilamide elixir) have caused drug safety to be a major point of concern to the FDA. All drugs are potentially harmful when taken at high dosage, and many have undesirable side effects. In this context, "safety" is assumed to imply an acceptably low risk of adverse effects with doses of the drug which provide the desired therapeutic effects. In addition, safety in special situations may be important. For example, guidelines have been developed to indicate the safety of drugs during pregnancy, by assigning drugs to FDA Pregnancy Class A, B, C, D, or X. Class A drugs appear to have no teratogenic effects; risk increases through classes B, C, and D; and class X drugs are contraindicated in pregnancy.

III. CONTROLLED SUBSTANCES

The FEDERAL CONTROLLED SUBSTANCES ACT of 1970 controls the distribution of drugs and other substances which have the potential to cause physical or psychological dependence, and which are often subject to abuse (alcohol is not included). Enforcement of this act is the responsibility of the DEA (Drug Enforcement Agency), a division of the Department of Justice. Prescribers must register with the DEA before they can prescribe controlled substances.

Schedule I drugs have no accepted medical use in the United States. Examples include heroin, LSD, marijuana, and mescaline.

Schedule II drugs include most of the narcotic analgesics, certain stimulants (e.g., amphetamines), and most short-acting barbiturates.

The most common Schedule III drugs are combinations of Schedule II narcotics with non-narcotic additives (e.g., codeine plus aspirin).

Schedule IV drugs include benzodiazepines, propoxyphene and related compounds, phenobarbital, and non-amphetamine diet preparations.

Schedule V drugs are most commonly codeine-containing cough preparations, or the antidiarrheal combination of diphenoxylate plus atropine.

Prescriptions for Schedule II drugs are non-refillable, and may not be prescribed over the phone except in emergency situations. Refill restrictions (no more than 5 times within 6 months) apply to drugs in schedules III and IV. Other restrictions may be added by state and local regulations.

REVIEW QUESTIONS

ONE BEST ANSWER

1. A drug which is contraindicated for use in pregnancy would be classified in FDA Pregnancy Class:

   A. I
   B. A
   C. V
   D. CP
   E. X

2. The Drug Enforcement Agency (DEA) is a division of the:

   A. Department of the Interior
   B. Department of Justice
   C. Department of Health and Human Services
   D. Bureau of Narcotics and Dangerous Drugs
   E. Bureau of Alcohol, Tobacco and Firearms

3. How many refills of prescriptions for schedule II controlled substances are allowed in the United States?

   A. None
   B. One only
   C. Three only
   D. Five, within 6 months of original filling of the prescription
   E. Federal law does not place limits on prescription refills

4. If a prescription is written for one teaspoonful of antibiotic suspension, to be taken four times a day for seven days, about what volume of suspension would be required?

   A. 100 ml
   B. 150 ml
   C. 200 ml
   D. 250 ml
   E. 300 ml

ANNOTATED ANSWERS TO REVIEW QUESTIONS

CHAPTER 1: GENERAL PRINCIPLES

1. __E__ Glutathione conjugation

2. __B__ Slow acetylators may accumulate isoniazid, hydralazine, and related aromatic amine drugs.

3. __D__ Induction involves increased expression of naturally occurring genes.

4. __E__ A is incorrect as antagonists do not increase drug effects. B defines a competitive-irreversible inhibitor which would give a similar change in dose-response curves. C is incorrect as dissociation constants for antagonists must be lower (higher affinity) than those for agonists. D is incorrect as spare receptors are an operational term and these do not differ from regular receptors. E is correct as these antagonists act at a site other than the binding site for the agonist to change its ability to interact with the receptor.

5. __B__ X_0 can be calculated from the data given. $t\frac{1}{2}$ is 4 hrs. Twice plasma concentration at 4 hrs is 4.8 µg/ml or 4.8 mg/L.

   $$V.D. = \frac{dose}{X_0} = \frac{500}{4.8} = \text{about 100 L}$$

6. __C__ Need to solve for dose in formula:

   $$\text{Plasma concentration} = \frac{1.5 \ (dose/interval)(t\frac{1}{2})}{vol. \ distribution}$$

   Toxic (4.5) - ineffective (2.0) = 2.5/2 = 1.3;
   2.0 + 1.3 = 3.3 µg/ml

   $$3.3 \ \text{µg/ml} = \frac{1.5 \ (D/8) \ (4)}{100L.}$$

   $$3.3 = \frac{0.75D}{100}$$

   = 440 mg

7. __B__ Variation equal to dose divided by volume of distribution.

8. __E__ $t\frac{1}{2} = 0.7 \ \dfrac{V.D.}{clearance}$

   $4 \ hr = 0.7 \ \dfrac{100 \ L}{clearance}$

   $Cl = \dfrac{70}{4}$ = about 18L/hr = 300 ml/min

   This clearance is greater than GFR but much less than renal plasma flow.

9. __C__ A is incorrect because there is not enough information available for this calculation. Drugs are compared for relative efficacy by calculating the percentage receptor occupation using the doses which produce a given equivalent response and the dissociation constants for the two drugs. C is the most correct answer here although it is really a suggestion; parallel curves do not prove that the drugs act at the same receptors; however, D is incorrect because if the curves are not parallel, the receptors can not be the same for the two responses. Drug A is more potent than Drug B as it causes the same effect at lower doses.

10. __A__ The certain safety factor is LD_1/ED_{99} and the curves for Drug B overlap substantially more than the curves for Drug A.

11. __E__ A is incorrect because converting to probits straightens the curve from a sigmoidal curve. Hyperbolas are seen with arithmetic doses and arithmetic responses on the X and Y axes respectively. B is incorrect because no manipulation can make those curves parallel. C is a question about relative efficacy and the calculation for that is given in the answer to question 9. D is incorrect as weak or partial agonists have to do with the requirement to fill all of the receptors to produce a maximal response and not the parallelism of dose-response curves. Tables for the conversion of responses to probits can be found in some texts.

12. __D__ A is incorrect because as more drug is available more is excreted and the plasma concentration of free drug will return to the previous steady-state and not maintain the increase. B is incorrect as the structural specificity for binding to plasma protein is much broader than that for a receptor; the two drugs may act at the same receptor but probably not. C is incorrect and the reasoning is like that given above for the response to answer A. E is incorrect as it is weak bases that bind to that plasma protein.

CHAPTER 1(Continued)

13. __D__ A is incorrect because this rate of infusion will not reach a toxic concentration even if continued longer; the final amount would be 450 mg. However, for some questions, this time is about 3 half-lives which would be slightly less than 90% of the final accumulation and this value can be used to calculate the amount present at that time. B is incorrect because the time to steady-state is dependent only on the half-life of the drug and not the dose. C is incorrect because at 3 hours the amount present would be 50% (450 mg) of the final accumulation (900 mg). Notice that doubling of the dose doubles the accumulation. An important point unrelated to this question is that doubling of the dose for drugs which follow first order kinetics will increase the duration of action by only one half-life. E is incorrect as these processes will eventually equal the rate of administration for any drug and more predictably with those which follow first order kinetics.

14. __C__ This question just involves following the drug concentrations through half-lives; starts at 450 mg, goes to 225 in one half-life, then 112 mg, then 56 mg.

15. __D__ A is incorrect as the large surface area, high blood flow and moderate pH present a favorable environment for absorption of both weak acids and weak bases. B is incorrect as some drugs are destroyed at low pH. E is incorrect as adsorption to food usually decrease absorption.

16. __D__ A is incorrect as penetration into the brain generally requires high lipid solubility which is also involved in fat storage. B is incorrect as binding to plasma protein is generally reversible. C is incorrect because different bonds are involved in binding to nucleic acids and fats. E is incorrect as binding to fat increases duration of action.

17. __B__ A is incorrect as these are strong agonists although Drug C is less potent than the other two agonists. C is incorrect as potency is not related to site of action. D is incorrect as the maximal response is decreased, the hallmark of receptor loss and not competition. Curve D is incorrect as the maximal response is indicating a lesser ability to cause a stimulus.

18. __D__ B is correct as no spare receptors are found for partial agonists. D is incorrect as spare receptors differ only from full receptors as a concept and not in the way they bind drugs or interact with second messenger systems.

19. __D__ A is incorrect because the clearance value is not high enough to indicate active secretion. B is incorrect because the large value for the volume of distribution indicates binding to tissue constituents which limits presentation of the drug to site of metabolism. C is incorrect because the calculated value is .001 /min. E is incorrect because the volume of distribution suggests, but does not prove, that the drug is lipid soluble and thus should pass through the blood-brain barrier.

20. __C__ A is correct as phorbol esters stimulate protein kinase C. B is correct as calmodulin bound with calcium activates a kinase. D is correct as the insulin receptor acts as a tyrosine kinase when activated. The nicotinic receptor can be phosphorylated but that event is not dependent directly on agonist binding.

21. __D__ A is incorrect because there are not sufficient free fatty acids present to influence pH; storage in fat is dependent on lipid solubility. B is incorrect because weak bases tend to be unionized in alkaline urine and thus reabsorbed. C is incorrect as both weak acids and weak bases are absorbed well in the small intestine because of the large surface area and high blood flow. E is incorrect as active secretion is not related to ion-trapping.

22. __D__ D is the exception as all lipid soluble substances penetrate the blood-brain barrier.

23. __C__ A is incorrect as covalent binding may occur with agents which are not classified as antagonists. B is incorrect as chemotherapeutic agents act through many mechanisms unrelated to covalent binding. E would be correct if the binding were confined to the receptor site alone but is not correct relative to binding in general.

CHAPTER 1 (Continued)

24. __D__ A is incorrect as intrinsic efficacy is an unknown property of the drug and clearly not related to the molecular weight. B is incorrect as there are several examples of receptors with multiple subunits. C is close but binding alone is not sufficient to identify the receptor. E is incorrect as the total number of receptors is an integral part of the kinetics of drug receptor interactions. The argument might be made that spare receptors negates this function, but the greater the total number of receptors, the lower the concentration at which a full agonist will demonstrate a response.

25. __C__ Inositol triphosphate interacts with a specific receptor on intracellular membranes to cause the release of stored calcium ion.

26. __A__ The sublingual route clearly bypasses the splanchnic circulation.

27. __C__ A is incorrect as the half-life is inconsistent with storage. B is incorrect as the liver is capable of rapid metabolism. D is incorrect as even though the half-life is short, an active transport process can strip drug from plasma protein in one pass. E is incorrect as the half-life is too short for the rate of glomerular filtration.

28. __D__ D is correct in that the binding of drug to plasma protein will transport the drug quickly to its site of excretion by active transport. E is incorrect as concentration of the urine occurs.

29. __D__ D is incorrect as spare receptors have no relationship to mechanisms of tolerance.

30. __B__ A is incorrect as the plasma concentration should be doubled. C is incorrect as the plasma concentration is consistent with zero order kinetics which should give the loss of a constant amount with time. D is incorrect as this is the unit for first order kinetics.

31. __E__ E is incorrect as metabolism by the liver completely bypasses the importance of the kidney. An exception to this would occur if there were the accumulation of a toxic metabolite which is normally excreted by the kidney.

32. __D__ D is incorrect as even though the maximal response to drugs A and C are markedly different, drug C has a lower ED_{50}.

33. __D__ A mixture of A and B should still produce a maximal response.

34. __D__ D is the exception as there are no real difference between "spare" receptors and regular receptors.

35. __A__

36. __C__

37. __B__ Zero order kinetics suggest that a drug is being metabolized and/or excreted as rapidly as the body is capable, so that competitive inhibition of metabolism may lead to accumulation of the drug.

38. __I__ Glucuronyltransferase

39. __H__ N-Acetyltransferase determines "rapid" or "slow" acetylators

40. __C__ Monoamine oxidase attacks the side chain

41. __E__ COMT methylate the catechol nucleus

42. __A__ CYP enzymes of different families are involved in glucocorticoid biosynthesis and drug metabolism, but several different isozymes are inhibited by metyrapone.

43. __G__ Accumulation of acetaldehyde after a drink of alcohol produces a variety of unpleasant symptoms.

44. __K__ Chloramphenicol sodium succinate is an ester for i.v. infusion, but esterases must release the parent compound. Similar reactions occur with esters of erythromycin and some cephalosporins.

45. __A__ Mixed function oxidase. Cytochrome P-450 is induced by phenobarbital (classical example) and many other drugs. However, phenobarbital also induces certain glucuronyltransferases (choice I) and glutathione S-transferases (choice J) enzymes; these choices are not "incorrect", but have little therapeutic significance.

46. __A__ Demethylation reactions are catalyzed by cytochrome P-450

47. __B__ Xanthine oxidase metabolizes purines and xanthines to urate derivatives.

48. __J__ Glutathione is a tripeptide of cysteine, glutamate and glycine.

49. __D__ Bacterial glucuronidases and sulfatases cleave corresponding conjugates. Reabsorption of the liberated parent drug completes "enterohepatic circulation".

50. __F__ Alcohol dehydrogenase. Aldehydes formed by this enzyme are converted to the corresponding acids by aldehyde dehydrogenases; patients develop metabolic acidosis from accumulation of formic acid (methanol) or glycolic acid (ethylene glycol).

CHAPTER 1 (Continued)

51. __A__ Malignant hyperthermia has been observed with both halothane and succinylcholine as well as other general anesthetic agents. Neuromuscular blocking drugs which stabilize the membrane potential have not been associated with this syndrome.

52. __D__

53. __C__

54. __B__ Induction of heme biosynthesis by barbiturates leads to increased porphyrin levels.

CHAPTER 2: DRUGS ACTING ON THE PERIPHERAL NERVOUS SYSTEM

1. __E__ Bethanechol is the drug of choice as acetylcholine is too short acting and methacholine produces intense cardiovascular (vasodilator) responses. The other agents (atropine and C_6 will decrease G.I. and bladder motility.

2. __E__ Acetylcholine is released at all ganglia (including the adrenal gland) and at the NMJ.

3. __E__ No single drug can produce miosis (increased parasympathetic mechanisms) and paralysis of accommodation (cycloplegia) due to blockade of cholinergic function.

4. __E__ NE would be expected to produce a reflex bradycardia. All of the drugs mentioned would prevent this reflex effect. Ganglionic block prevents reflexes; muscarinic blockade would eliminate the vagal input of the heart; α-adrenoceptor blockade would prevent the vasoconstrictor action of NE.

5. __C__ Only an anticholinesterase drug which would increase the effective levels of ACh at autonomic parasympathetic postganglionic synapses would cause all of these physiological responses.

6. __E__ Atracurium is the choice as all of the other drugs are eliminated by either metabolic or renal routes.

7. __A__ Succinylcholine causes depolarization blockade at the NMJ endplate, thus the increased effective level of ACh at this synapse would enhance the extent of blockade. Neostigmine might be used to reverse the skeletal muscle blocking actions of the competitive blockers (e.g., B, C and D). Hemicholinium results in depletion of transmitter by preventing uptake of choline.

8. __A__ The parasympathetic ganglia to the heart are so close to the tissue that vagal nerve stimulations must always be preganglionic. Thus, atropine and ganglionic blockers will prevent this activation.

9. __B__ Clonidine is an α_2-adrenoceptor stimulant and yohimbine is an α_2-adrenoceptor antagonist. All of the other drugs act on ß-adrenoceptors.

10. __E__ Although the precise reason is not known, timolol is unique among the ß-adrenoceptor antagonists listed in that it acts potently in the eye to suppress formation of aqueous humor. Yohimbine is an α_2-adrenoceptor blocker with little effect on aqueous pressure.

11. __C__ MAO in the CNS mainly produces the phenylglycol. In peripheral nerves the most common metabolite is the mandelic acid.

12. __D__ The side effects mentioned are characteristic of α-adrenoceptor blockade (e.g., phenoxybenzamine).

13. __D__ Reserpine depletes nerve endings of catecholamines. Thus, those drugs that act "indirectly" to release stored NE will not be as active after reserpine pretreatment (e.g. methamphetamine, tyramine, and ephedrine). Prazosin administration lowers blood pressure by blocking tonic release of NE. If the nerves are depleted of NE, then there is nothing further for prazosin to antagonize. Methoxamine is a direct acting sympathomimetic which will still vasoconstrict after reserpine.

14. __A__ Norepinephrine action will be seen only on α-adrenoceptors as the ß-adrenoceptors are antagonized by propranolol. Thus you will not observe an action to increase heart rate. Stimulation of both α- and ß-adrenoceptors acts to decrease tone of the G.I. smooth muscle.

15. __B__ Bronchial smooth muscle is relaxed by drugs or epinephrine acting on β_2-adrenoceptors. These would be blocked by propranolol.

16. __C__ Prazosin is a selective α_1-adrenoceptor antagonist. It is neither indirect acting nor is it a sympathomimetic.

17. __C__ Imipramine is a tricyclic antidepressant drug that acts to prevent reuptake of several monoamines including NE. Tyramine causes NE release; pargyline is a MAO inhibitor; prazosin and ritodrine act directly to block or stimulate specific adrenergic receptors.

CHAPTER 2 (Continued)

18. _E_ Metoprolol is a ß-adrenoceptor antagonist. All of the others would stimulate ß-adrenoceptors.

19. _C_ Although all of the choices for drug X would lower blood pressure, only the ß-adrenoceptor stimulant isoproterenol would not be antagonized by the respective drug Y (scopolamine is a muscarinic receptor antagonist).

20. _D_ Phenylephrine is an α-adrenoceptor stimulant. The large rise in blood pressure causes a potent baroreceptor reflex causing increase vagal tone to slow the heart and also withdrawal of sympathetic neural tone to the heart.

21. _B_ Amphetamine acts mainly to release NE from nerve endings (and to some extent prevents reuptake) thus is classified as an "indirect" sympathomimetic.

22. _E_ NE, EPI, and ISO are catecholamines with OHs on benzine ring and no protection of the terminal nitrogen with a C_3 moiety on the α-carbon (thus they would be inactivated by both COMT and MAO). Hexamethonium is highly charged and not orally efficacious. Ephedrine is protected from MAO breakdown and has no OHs on benzine ring for COMT action.

23. _E_ Epinephrine causes bronchiolar smooth muscle relaxation, not constriction.

24. _B_ Although some of the other reasons are true or partially so, only answer B is causally related to the statement.

25. _C_ An indirect acting sympathomimetic drug will release (or prevent reuptake) of catecholamines which act on both α- and ß-adrenoceptors. Thus, one would need both an α-adrenoceptor blocker (e.g., phenoxybenzamine) and a ß-adrenoceptor antagonist (e.g., propranolol).

26. _E_ The sequence of NE synthesis is: phenylalanine → tyrosine → DOPA → dopamine → NE. VMA is the major metabolite found in the urine after both COMT and MAO have degraded NE.

27. _D_ Contraction of the radial muscle of the iris results in mydriasis. This is mediated via α adrenergic receptors (i.e., blocked by phenoxybenzamine and phentolamine but not by propranolol).

28. _C_ Atropine administration causes mydriasis or dilation of the pupil in that the predominant parasympathetic tone is blocked. This might precipitate or worsen glaucoma. Atropine would have little if any effect in the other conditions mentioned.

29. _D_ Remember that the adrenergic receptors that NE acts on are α in the vasculature and ß in the heart. Thus the only agent that would produce the above mentioned effects would be an α blocker (e.g., prazosin).

30. _C_ Neostigmine complexes with the enzyme which breaks down ACh thus increases its effectiveness and duration at the NMJ. Remember that neostigmine also has a direct stimulation action on the postsynaptic receptors. Thus it has a dual effect, and consequently, is a drug of choice in treating myasthenia gravis. Motor nerve terminals are pre-synaptic.

31. _B_ This patient is most likely to have myasthenia gravis. If he already has a deficit in neuromuscular function, a competitive blocker like tubocurarine would be effective at lower doses than would be expected in the normal individual.

32. _B_ Pilocarpine is a muscarinic stimulant. It increases outflow of aqueous humor from the eye by constricting the pupil and contracting the ciliary muscle; the subsequent tension opens the outflow channels in the trabecular network.

33. _C_ Guanethidine would decrease release of NE from nerve endings thus potentially causing the receptors to become supersensitive to a direct acting sympathomimetic drug.

34. _B_ Carbachol would stimulate autonomic ganglia and the adrenal gland. Since both the non-innervated muscarinic receptors and the innervated α receptors on blood vessels are blocked, the circulating epinephrine from the adrenal gland would act on the non-innervated ß receptors to produce vasodilation and a lowering of blood pressure.

35. _A_ The nerve activity would increase due to both the direct ganglionic action of carbachol as well as the reflex compensation due to decreased blood pressure.

36. _A_

37. _D_ Don't confuse this drug with dopamine.

38. _B_ Only a ganglionic blocking agent will lower blood pressure as parasympathetic nerves do not innervate most blood vessels.

CHAPTER 2 (Continued)

39. __D__ Atropine enters CNS to produce excitation (others are quaternary ammonium agents).

40. __D__ Epinephrine acts on both α- and β_2-adrenoceptors to raise and lower blood pressure respectively. ß-Adrenoceptor blockade with nadolol would increase the α-adrenoceptor effect of Epi as it is no longer opposed by the vasodilator effect. The isoproterenol ß-adrenoceptor vasodilation would be blocked by nadolol.

41. __C__ All changes in blood pressure are buffered by baroreceptor reflexes tending to minimize the change. Hexamethonium will eliminate the efferent (motor) limb of the reflex and thus both elevations and reduction of pressure will be increased (enhanced).

42. __D__ Physostigmine is the most rational treatment. It enters the CNS and increases ACh levels to compete with the atropine.

43. __A__

44. __E__ Neostigmine not only is an anticholinesterase drug but will also act directly on skeletal muscle to enhance contractility.

45. __C__

46.-48. Reserpine will deplete the nerve ending of monoamines (e.g., NE). Thus, the effect of a mixed acting sympathomimetic will be reduced (ephedrine) and the actions of an indirect acting sympathomimetic (tyramine) would be lost. A direct acting sympathomimetic (methoxamine) would be the same or potentiated due to either supersensitivity and/or lowering of the initial starting blood pressure level.

46. __D__
47. __A__
48. __B__
49. __A__
50. __C__
51. __E__
52. __D__
53. __B__
54. __D__
55. __G__
56. __B__
57. __E__
58. __J__
59. __F__
60. __C__
61. __I__
62. __A__

63. __H__

64.-68. Phenylephrine will increase blood pressure by direct α-adrenoceptor stimulation. The response in these nerves to increased pressure is to increase firing in the carotid sinus afferent nerves which excites vagal outflow and inhibits the sympathetic efferent outflow to the blood vessels and heart as in question #64. In question #65, the answer will be the same because depletion of NE by reserpine would only augment the pressor action of phenylephrine. In #66, hexamethonium (C_6) will block efferent ganglionic transmission, thus no activity is possible in the post-ganglionic nerves. In #67, phenoxybenzamine will prevent the pressor effect of phenylephrine, thus no change in blood pressure and no change in firing of nerves. The final question (#68) demonstrates that the neural response to carotid occlusion still occurs even though the blood pressure does not change due to blockade of all relevant end organs.

64. __B__
65. __B__
66. __E__
67. __A__
68. __D__

69-72. In #69, when nicotine is given i.v. the first organ to see the drug is the heart where parasympathetic ganglia are located in the muscle wall. Then as the nicotine is pumped around it can then activate the sympathetic ganglia and adrenal gland. This provides the biphasic response shown. Reserpine eliminates the pressor response; atropine blocks the depressor response caused by severe slowing of heart rate. In #70, drug B must be a direct acting sympathomimetic (alpha) as effect is potentiated by amine depletion. Ephedrine would be partially reduced in effect by depletion as about half of its actions are indirect (release of NE from nerve endings). In #71, drug C must be an indirect acting sympathomimetic as the action is blocked by depletion of NE with reserpine. In #72, drug D is blocked by atropine. Pilocarpine acts on non-innervated muscarinic receptors of vasculature causing vasodilation.

69. __A__
70. __E__
71. __B__
72. __C__

CHAPTER 2 (Continued)

73. - 80. First look at over-all problem and note that all effects are eventually blocked. As there is no angiotensin receptor blocker in the pretreatment group you can discard angiotensin as a potential answer. Pressor drugs (A and C) could be either tyramine or norepinephrine (NE). Depressor drugs are either acetylcholine (ACh) or methacholine. As drug B is blocked and the large dose of ACh shows reversal of action (depressor to pressor) the only possible answer is drug B = methacholine and drug D = ACh and blocker P = atropine. The reversal of ACh after atropine is a ganglionic stimulating effect, thus pretreatment Q must be the ganglionic blocker hexamethonium. With regard to the two pressor drugs, depletion of the endogenous stores of NE would selectively prevent the actions of the indirect sympathomimetic, tyramine. α-Adrenoceptor blockade would block both NE and tyramine. Thus agonist A is tyramine and R is reserpine. Agonist C is NE which is blocked by pretreatment S, phenoxybenzamine.

73. __C__
74. __B__
75. __D__
76. __A__
77. __A__
78. __D__
79. __B__
80. __C__

CHAPTER 3: DRUGS ACTING ON THE KIDNEY

1. __B__ Desmopressin
2. __E__ Thiazide diuretics
3. __D__ Lithium carbonate
4. __B__ The most effective diuretics (urine volume) and natriuretics (sodium excretion) inhibit chloride absorption in the ascending loop of Henle. An example of a loop diuretic is furosemide.
5. __D__ Triamterene directly inhibits sodium/potassium exchange in the distal convoluted tubule. Sodium is excreted and potassium is retained. The remaining diuretic agents increase sodium delivery to the distal convoluted tubule and thereby stimulate sodium/potassium exchange, resulting in increased potassium excretion (hypokalemia)

6. __C__ Acetazolamide will increase uric acid excretion by alkalinizing the urine. The thiazide and loop diuretics all decrease uric acid excretion by inhibiting the active secretion of uric acid in the proximal convoluted tubule.
7. __D__ Mannitol is an osmotic agent which increases urine volume (increases water excretion) without altering sodium reabsorption. a, b, c, and e increase both sodium and water excretion
8. __L__ Acetazolamide
9. __B__ Triamterene
10. __H__ Hydrochlorothiazide
11. __E__ Propranolol
12. __J__ Captopril
13. __D__ Spironolactone
14. __J__ Captopril
15. __L__ Acetazolamide
16. __H__ Hydrochlorothiazide
17. __H__ Hydrochlorothiazide
18. __F__ Acetazolamide

CHAPTER 4: DRUGS ACTING ON THE CARDIOVASCULAR SYSTEM

1. __E__ Propranolol (a beta-adrenergic receptor antagonist) does not alter smooth muscle tone in large coronary arteries. Both organic nitrates and calcium antagonists prevent/reverse coronary artery spasm.
2. __D__ Although quinidine produces some slowing of AV conduction via a direct blockade of sodium ion channels, quinidine is also an anticholinergic drug, and will facilitate conduction through the AV node by blocking the actions of the vagus nerve.
3. __D__ The duration of the QT interval is determined by action potential duration in ventricular myocardium. Mexiletine, and all other Class IB antiarrhythmic drugs, shorten action potential duration. Class IA drugs increase action potential duration and Class IC drugs do not alter action potential duration.
4. __E__ Verapamil is the calcium entry blocker which produces the greatest depression of AV nodal function, sinus nodal function, and myocardial contractility.
5. __D__ Nifedipine reduces myocardial oxygen consumption via a dramatic decrease in afterload and a smaller decrease in preload

CHAPTER 4 (Continued)

6. __C__ Propranolol decreases myocardial oxygen consumption by producing dramatic decreases in the sinus heart rate and myocardial contractility. Both changes results from beta-adrenergic receptor blockade. The drug also mildly increases preload and afterload, somewhat reducing the previously noted beneficial actions of the drug.

7. __C__

8. __C__

9. __A__

10. __D__ Plasma renin levels would increase in response to decreased perfusion pressure of kidney, decreased sympathetic tone or due to Na⁺ loss. Alpha-methyldopa would decrease sympathetic tone to kidney thus inhibit neural renin release. The beta blockers would block the renal receptors activated by sympathetic tone to kidney.

11. __D__ Blood pressure in a patient with congestive failure is usually about normal or a bit on the low side, depending upon the severity of the failure and the degree of compensation. Digitalis, because of the improved cardiac output, will improve hemodynamics and return pressure towards normal; it definitely will not fall.

12. __D__ When effective refractory period is prolonged, fewer impulses can pass through the node and ventricular rate is slowed.

13. __E__ Digitalis enhances vagal tone to the sinus node by several mechanisms and will slow the discharge of impulses from the node. Thus, sinus bradycardia is the result unless vagal tone is already high; in this case, heart rate may not change.

14. __B__ Glycosides are most effective in low output failure; they are ineffective in high output failure or if myocardial damage results from a toxic process.

15. __B__ Glycosides enhance vagal tone to the AV node to slow conduction of impulses through the node. The P-R interval is an index of AV conduction time. Since AV conduction time is longer, P-R interval is prolonged.

16. __D__

17. __D__ The therapeutic and toxic effects of cardiac glycosides are closely linked to extracellular potassium. Although toxicity would be decreased by raising serum K⁺, the therapeutic effect also would be decreased.

18. __C__ Digoxin has a half-life of about 1.5 days; digitoxin has the long half-life.

19. __D__ Cholestyramine is a non-absorbed ion-exchange resin that binds bile acids in the gut. It does not affect the biosynthesis of cholesterol.

20. __E__ Nicotinamide is interchangeable with nicotinic acid as a vitamin but has none of the effects of nicotinic acid to lower lipids

21. __C__
22. __D__
23. __A__
24. __B__
25. __E__
26. __C__
27. __B__
28. __D__
29. __E__
30. __F__
31. __A__
32. __A__
33. __C__
34. __B__
35. __G__
36. __F__
37. __B__ Nifedipine
38. __G__ Procainamide
39. __G__ Procainamide
40. __C__ Furosemide
41. __A__ Amiodarone
42. __C__ Furosemide
43. __D__ Flecainide is the best answer although congestive heart failure occurs with a lesser incidence with (E) Quinidine, (I) Verapamil, and (J) Procainamide
44. __A__ Amiodarone
45. __D__ Spironolactone
46. __J__ Lisinopril
47. __C__ Bretylium
48. __F__ Disopyramide
49. __G__ Flecainide
50. __O__ Diltiazem
51. __E__ Propranolol
52. __K__ Lidocaine
53. __D__ Nitroglycerin
54. __O__ Diltiazem (nifedipine is not an acceptable answer as the drug acts preferentially upon vascular smooth muscle)
55. __F__ Disopyramide
56. __E__ Propranolol
57. __H__ Hydrochlorothiazide
58. __E__ Propranolol

CHAPTER 5: DRUGS AFFECTING HEMOSTASIS AND HEMATOPOIESIS

1. __C__ Cobalamin (vitamin B_{12}). During the process of digestion and absorption, folates become methylated to biologically inactive products. These methyl groups are removed in a vitamin B_{12} dependent step, but methylated intermediates accumulate if there is a vitamin B_{12} deficiency.
2. __B__ Anemia associated with renal failure
3. __D__ Cobalamin (vitamin B_{12}).
4. __F__ Protamine
5. __B__ Vitamin K
6. __H__ Pentoxifyllin
7. __D__ Desmopressin
8. __G__ Heparin. Enoxaparin is also rapidly active, but its shorter chain gives it appreciable activity only against clotting factor Xa.
9. __I__ Streptokinase
10. __A__ Aminocaproic acid and tranhexamic acid antagonize actions of all the thrombolytic agents.
11. __K__ Tissue plasminogen activator
12. __J__ Sulfinpyrazone
13. __B__ These toxicities may occur with indanedione derivatives, but not with warfarin
14. __F__ Enoxaparin

CHAPTER 6: DRUGS ACTING ON THE CENTRAL NERVOUS SYSTEM

1. __C__ Opioids should not be used routinely as sedatives UNLESS the patient cannot sleep because they are in pain. There are safer and more effective agents currently available for use as sedatives.
2. __A__ Dull, constant pain has been shown to be better relieved than sharp, stabbing pain. As a result, opioid analgesics particularly are suited to treat chronic types of pain.
3. __A__ Naloxone undergoes significant first pass metabolism and as a result, is effective only when given by the intravenous route. Naloxone has a high affinity for mu receptors, it acts by competitive inhibition, will not worsen the respiratory depression caused by barbiturates and has a shorter half-life than morphine.
4. __B__ Minimal or no tolerance develops to the miosis and constipation produced by opioids.
5. __C__ The MAC is an ED50 value and gives an indication of the anesthetic potency.

6. __D__
7. __D__ Nitrous oxide is relatively insoluble in the blood; as a result, it has a rapid induction rate and a rapid recovery rate.
8. __D__ Pro-opiomelanocortin gives rise to the endorphins, not the enkephalins. The precursor for met- and leu-enkephalin is proenkephalin A.
9. __D__ An "ideal" anesthetic produces muscle relaxation, analgesia and unconsciousness. Most anesthetic agents are NOT ideal anesthetics; as a result, preoperative medications are administered with the primary anesthetic.
10. __C__ Local anesthetics block the propagation of nerve impulses along axons. NSAIDS block the initiation of pain impulses in the periphery and opioid analgesics inhibit the release of neurotransmitters from primary afferents in the spinal cord and the processing of painful information in the thalamus.
11. __B__ Halothane produces a dose-dependent hypotension; as a result, blood pressure should be monitored continuously.
12. __D__ Nitrous oxide is a relatively insoluble anesthetic. Upon termination of the anesthetic, the gas rushes back into the alveoli. This phenomenon is known as diffusion hypoxia and oxygen must be administered during this time to provide adequate oxygenation.
13. __B__ Many different types of agents with varied structures can produce general anesthesia. As a result, general anesthetics likely do not produce their effects by acting at specific receptor sites. It has been hypothesized that general anesthetics disrupt membrane structure and function to produce their effects.
14. __C__
15. __D__ The postoperative urinary retention produced by opioids is a peripheral action on the urethral sphincter.
16. __E__ All of the following factors listed influence the rate of induction of inhalation anesthetics.
17. __B__ Malignant hyperthermia is believed to be due to a massive release of Ca^{++} from the sarcoplasmic reticulum. Dantrolene prevents this Ca^{++} release.
18. __C__
19. __A__
20. __B__ Vasoconstrictors are added to local anesthetics to decrease systemic absorption and prolong the duration of action.

CHAPTER 6 (Continued)

21. __D__ Benzocaine is poorly water soluble, and as a result is only used as a topical local anesthetic.

22. __C__ Opioids have peripheral effects on the gastrointestinal tract which cause constipation as a side effect.

23. __B__ Local anesthetic agents can produce central nervous system effects if blood levels of the anesthetic are excessive. To minimize systemic absorption, local anesthetics often are administered with vasoconstrictors.

24. __E__ Codeine acts in the central nervous system to produce analgesia and aspirin acts peripherally to produce analgesia; as a result, the two agents' effects are additive. Pharmacologically it doesn't make sense to combine two agents with the same mechanisms of action (e.g., aspirin + acetaminophen), since no greater effect is achieved.

25. __B__ Enflurane should be used with caution in patients with a history of seizures.

26. __E__

27. __E__

28. __C__ Potency. These compounds are very similar in their actions. An effective dose of LSD is 25 µg, psilocybin 4 mg, and mescaline 0.2 g.

29. __B__ Sedation. With increasing doses of benzodiazepines there is progression from sedation to anaesthesia and coma. The sedation with antipsychotics is more of a state of indifference or apathy, with a drowsy feeling and motor inactivity, but they can be aroused. Benzodiazepines, but not phenothiazines, produce physical dependence and have muscle-relaxant activity; phenothiazines produce extrapyramidal symptoms, tremors and spastic movements, and some of the phenothiazines are potent antiemetics.

30. __C__ The central depressant actions of the barbiturates are terminated by three mechanisms: very short acting-very lipid soluble compounds, such as thiopental, by physical redistribution; short and intermediate acting compounds, such as pentobarbital, by metabolism--generally to a hydroxylated compound, and long acting-low lipid soluble compounds, by renal excretion as well as by metabolism.

31. __B__

32. __D__ MPTP was a by-product in the illicit manufacture of meperidine. MPTP is a protoxin taken up by astrocytes and metabolized by MAO to a stable charged ion that selectively damages striatal dopaminergic neurons. Ecstasy (MDMA) is reported in animals to destroy serotonergic neurons.

33. __D__

34. __B__ Methylphenidate is preferred to dextroamphetamine because it has equal efficacy without long term inhibition of growth.

35. __D__

36. __A__ Procyclidine is used for rigidity, trihexyphenidyl or benztropine is used for tremor, and if bradykinesia is present, either amantadine or L-DOPA is used.

37. __C__

38. __B__ The fused triazolo ring prevents the formation of desmethylbenzodiazepine. Triazolam and alprazolam form an alpha hydroxylated metabolite which is pharmacologically inactive. The difference between triazolam and alprazolam is that triazolam is marketed exclusively as a hypnotic while alprazolam is marketed for anxiety particularly with depression.

39. __D__ Malnutrition. Remember that malnutrition is not only caused by inadequate dietary intake but also by GI absorption impairment, pancreatic insufficiently, defective cofactors for metabolism, and storage of nutrients.

40. __D__

41. __C__ Saturation of metabolic pathways occurs in the therapeutic range; phenytoin follows Michaelis-Menten kinetics rather than first order or zero order kinetics.

42. __B__

43. __C__ Haloperidol is almost always the antipsychotic drug used for novel or acute conditions. Ballismus is the result of acute vascular infarctions of the subthalamic nucleus of Luysii. Prognosis is grave without immediate pharmacological treatment.

44. __B__

45. __D__

46. __D__ The piperidine side chain phenothiazines (thioridazine) have no clinical efficacy as antiemetics in man. Promethazine is not an antipsychotic phenothiazine (only two carbon bridge) but it is an effective antiemetic because of its cholinergic blocking activity.

CHAPTER 6 (Continued)

47. __D__ Although renal tubular necrosis and diabetes insipidus are chronic toxicities of lithium the incidence is rare.
48. __C__ Withdrawal will produce insomnia.
49. __D__ Meperidine is a opioid analgesic; secobarbital and alcohol are sedative-hypnotics. Both classes produce physical dependence and marked withdrawal. Marihuana does not produce physical dependence; there are no consistent withdrawal signs or symptoms.
50. __D__ While tolerance will develop at a different rate for different opioid analgesics, it always develops faster at higher doses with a frequent dosing schedule. Obviously if the dose is small enough and over an extended time period no tolerance will occur. Tolerance does not develop at the same rate for all actions. Little tolerance occurs to the constipating, miotic and cortex-spinal stimulating effects. Tolerance develops quickly to respiratory depression, tolerance develops slightly slower to the euphoria and analgesia. Cross tolerance exists between the opioid analgesics. Disappearance of tolerance also has a variable course.
51. __D__ Buspirone is an anxiolytic agent that does not produce muscle relaxation or have other properties of sedative-hypnotic drugs. Phenobarbital is seldom prescribed but could be used.
52. __A__ These effects generally increase during dosage regulation due to excessive dopamine in the brain.
53. __C__ Treatment is the same as for Parkinson's disease. Haloperidol is a dopamine antagonist.
54. __A__
55. __B__ Clomipramine is effective is about 50-70% of the patients while imipramine and diazepam are effective in 5% or less.
56. __D__ The first three foils are the criteria to obtain rapid onset. Foil 4 is of importance for the duration of action.
57. __B__ Diarrhea can occur later in the withdrawal process.
58. __E__
59. __E__ Ethanol absorption is virtually 100% from the GI tract. The amount of ethanol expired in the breath is negligible, and urinary loss is only about 5%.
60. __B__ Ketamine
61. __B__ Sumatripan

62. __E__ Dihydroergotamine
63. __C__ Caffeine
64. __D__ Methysergide
65. __F__ Carbamazepine
66. __L__ Flumazenil
67. __Z__ Selegiline
68. __R__ LSD
69. __G__ Clozapine
70. __T__ Marihuana
71. __N__ Fluorothyl
72. __U__ Midazolam
73. __X__ Pimozide
74. __W__ Phencyclidine
75. __Y__ Procyclidine
76. __Q__ Loxapine
77. __D__ Bupropion
78. __S__ Maprotiline
79. __H__ Cyclobenzaprine
80. __B__ Baclofen
81. __C__ Buprenorphine
82. __D__ Bupropion

CHAPTER 7: AUTACOIDS AND THE THERAPY OF INFLAMMATION

1. __E__ The hepatotoxicity in acetaminophen overdose is produced by a toxic metabolite.
2. __D__ NSAIDs do not have significant effects on the respiratory system at therapeutic doses; this represents one of the main advantages of NSAIDs over opioid analgesics.
3. __E__
4. __C__
5. __D__
6. __B__ The sedative effects produced by some H_1 antihistamines can limit their therapeutic usefulness; newer antihistamines have been developed that are non-sedating.
7. __D__ Renin converts angiotensinogen to angiotensin I.
8. __B__
9. __B__
10. __A__ Bradykinin is a potent constrictor of uterine, bronchiolar and gastrointestinal smooth muscle.
11. __B__
12. __E__
13. __B__ The oxicams are a new class of NSAIDs; their primary advantage is pharmacokinetic in nature. They have a half-life of approx. 50 hrs which allows for single daily dosing. This is an important factor for patients who must take these agents on a chronic, long-term basis.

CHAPTER 7 (Continued)

14. __D__ Gold salts may induce partial or complete remission of rheumatoid arthritis; the duration of the remission is variable and the mechanism by which the remission is produced is unknown.

15. __C__

16. __B__ Aspirin does not lower body temperature in non-febrile patients and aspirin toxicity is associated with hyperthermia.

17. __A__

18. __B__ Initially aspirin toxicity produces respiratory alkalosis; this is followed by respiratory and metabolic acidosis.

19. __D__

20. __B__

21. __C__ H_2 antihistamines are therapeutically used to treat duodenal and gastric ulcers.

22. __E__

23. __B__ Antihistamines are relatively ineffective in the treatment of anaphylactoid reactions.

24. __B__ Serotonin's primary effect is vasoconstriction of most arteries, veins and venules which results in increased blood pressure.

25. __C__ Methysergide inhibits the vasoconstrictor and pressor effects produced by serotonin and is used prophylactically to treat migraines.

26. __B__

27. __C__

28. __B__

29. __D__ Sulfinpyrazone is a uricosuric agent and does not produce its effects by interfering with prostaglandin synthesis.

30. __C__

31. __B__

32. __A__ H_1 antihistamine

33. __H__ Terfenadine poorly penetrates the CNS and is a non-sedating H_1 antihistamine.

34. __O__ Inhibits the release of histamine from mast cells in the lung; is only useful prophylactically for asthma treatment.

35. __C__ H_2 antihistamine; inhibits gastric secretions.

36. __I__ Potent antihistamine and antiserotonin agent.

37. __Q__ Inhibits the vasoconstrictor and pressor effects produced by serotonin.

38. __E__

39. __G__ Acetaminophen is the drug of choice since aspirin causes an increased incidence of Reye's syndrome in children with influenza or chicken pox.

40. __M__ Angiotensin converting enzyme inhibitor.

41. __B__ PGE_2 prostaglandin

42. __L__ Inactivates the toxic metabolite; must be given within 10-24 hrs of overdose.

CHAPTER 8: THE ENDOCRINE SYSTEM

1. __C__

2. __D__

3. __A__ B is correct but does not explain the mechanism of action.

4. __D__

5. __C__ One or two large doses have no adverse effects. Treatment of the other conditions require chronic dosing schedules.

6. __D__

7. __E__ A is incorrect as sodium ion is lost in the diuresis. B is one of the actions of insulin. C is incorrect as 2,3-diphosphoglycerate is decreased in RBCs limiting oxygen release. D is incorrect as acidosis subsequent to insulin deficiency should increase this ratio.

8. __E__

9. __A__

10. __E__

11. __D__

12. __D__

13. __E__ Methylprednisolone does not have much influence on mineral balance. A mineralocorticoid would cause hypernatremia and hypokalemia.

14. __D__

15. __B__ Parenteral testosterone esters are preferred for long-term use because they are more effective and they lack the hepatotoxicity of 17 α-alkylated compounds.

16. __B__

17. __D__

18. __A__

19. __C__

20. __D__ Vasopressin is a vasoconstrictor; oxytocin is a vasodilator.

21. __E__ Oxytocin stimulates milk letdown (or ejection) in nursing mothers, but not milk "production".

22. __C__ One of the most important actions of insulin is its ability to inhibit glucose production by the liver.

CHAPTER 8 (Continued)

23. __C__ A is incorrect as the complex is insoluble and should not be given I.V. B is incorrect as the preparation has all the properties associated with regular insulin as far as effects on metabolism. E is incorrect as hypoglycemia is the most prevalent toxicity of insulin no matter the route of administration or the preparation.

24. __B__ A is incorrect as both agents are ineffective in IDDM. C and E are true of both agents.

25. __E__ E is the exception as the toxicity would be hypercalcemia.

26. __E__ A is correct as exercise increases glucose utilization by a mechanism which is not dependent on insulin. E is the exception as an α-adrenergic blocking drug does not have a documented interaction with insulin in the diabetic patient.

27. __A__
28. __C__
29. __B__
30. __B__
31. __D__
32. __E__
33. __A__ Remember that estrogen withdrawal can cause menstruation
34. __C__
35. __B__
36. __C__
37. __A__
38. __E__
39. __C__ Intermediate-duration glucocorticoids are often used for alternate day therapy
40. __B__
41. __E__
42. __D__
43. __A__ Hydrocortisone is preferred because of its salt-retaining activity

CHAPTER 9: ANTI-INFECTIVE AGENTS

1. __C__ Doxycycline
2. __A__ Aztreonam
3. __D__ Clavulanic acid
4. __D__ Lincomycin is poorly absorbed
5. __B__ Order is reversed for gram positive
6. __A__ Amikacin
7. __E__ Nystatin
8. __D__ Sulfadiazine
9. __B__ Sulfasalazine
10. __A__ Chloramphenicol
11. __C__ Dicloxacillin

12. __D__ Aztreonam
13. __D__ Sulfamethoxazole and trimethoprim inhibit bacterial folic acid metabolism at two different steps. Clavulanic acid is synergistic with ticarcillin because it inhibits beta-lactamase. Mandelic acid acidifies the urine and optimizes the activity of methenamine. Ampicillin and gentamicin have different, but complimentary, mechanisms of action.
14. __A__ Azithromycin
15. __D__ Amantadine is not metabolized.
16. __D__ Acyclovir. Toxicity is much greater for the virus than for the host because the activity of acyclovir depends on its intracellular phosphorylation to acycloGMP by a virus-encoded thymidine kinase and because viral DNA polymerase is more sensitive to inhibition by acycloGTP than is mammalian DNA polymerase.
17. __B__
18. __A__
19. __D__ Zidovudine inhibits reverse transcriptase, but it also incorporates into viral DNA and causes chain termination.
20. __A__ AZT produces anemia and neutropenia but rarely thrombocytopenia.
21. __D__
22. __E__
23. __G__ Reverse transcriptase is an RNA-dependent, DNA polymerase.
24. __A__
25. __C__
26. __K__ See Chapter 10
27. __D__
28. __J__
29. __B__
30. __H__
31. __F__
32. __I__ See Chapter 10
33. __C__ Rocky Mountain Spotted Fever is a rickettsial infection, treated preferably with a tetracycline. Chloramphenicol is an alternate drug from the list given.
34. __D__ Salmonella species are resistant to most antibiotics, but chloramphenicol is usually effective. Some Salmonella respond to third generation cephalosporins, so ceftazidime is a potential alternate drug.
35. __L__ Penetration across the blood-brain barrier is a special property of fluconazole.

CHAPTER 9 (Continued)

36. _F_ Erythromycin is usually listed as the drug of choice for Legionnaires's Disease, but clarithromycin generally has a lower MIC value.
37. _G_ Many strains of Staphylococci produce penicillinase, and often a penicillinase-resistant penicillin is recommended to initiate therapy.
38. _I_ Dapsone
39. _H_ Pseudomonal infections are often treated with a third generation cephalosporin, possibly in combination with an aminoglycoside. Ceftazidime has the highest anti-Pseudomonal activity among the cephalosporins.
40. _K_ One-dose treatment of gonorrhea is the only indication for spectinomycin.
41. _E_ Rifampin is the only drug listed with substantial anti-tubercular activity
42. _B_ Clindamycin is effective for most anaerobic infections, and is usually considered the drug of choice for Bacteroides.
43. _J_ Vancomycin is indicated for methicillin-resistant Staphylococci.
44. _C_
45. _D_
46. _A_
47. _E_
48. _B_
49. _B_
50. _D_
51. _A_
52. _E_
53. _C_

CHAPTER 10: CANCER CHEMOTHERAPY AND IMMUNOSUPPRESSIVE AGENTS

1. _D_ Busulfan
2. _A_ Azathioprine
3. _D_ Methotrexate
4. _B_ Mechlorethamine is too reactive to be useful as an immunosuppressant
5. _C_ Etoposide
6. _B_
7. _D_ Bleomycin
8. _B_
9. _D_ Mercaptopurine
10. _C_ Doxorubicin
11. _A_ Vincristine
12. _B_ Cyclophosphamide

13. _E_ Tamoxifen
14. _D_ Methotrexate
15. _A_ Mercaptopurine
16. _C_ Doxorubicin
17. _B_ Vinblastine
18. _C_ Daunorubicin
19. _B_ Leuprolide
20. _D_ Bleomycin
21. _A_ Vincristine
22. _E_ Carmustine

CHAPTER 11: CHEMOTHERAPY OF PARASITIC DISEASES

1. _B_ The correct answer is metronidazole, which is preferred over the others because it is considered less toxic.
2. _B_ The correct answer is chloroquine, which is ineffective against colonic infections. For this reason a drug effective against intestinal amebiasis (metronidazole) is preferred.
3. _D_ The correct answer is metronidazole. Dehydroemetine does not eradicate cysts. Chloroquine is concentrated in the liver and is intestinally ineffective. Iodoquinol is effective in the cyst passing patient but much less effective in acute dysentery.
4. _C_ The correct answer is diloxanide, which is effective administered alone in eliminating cysts.
5. _C_ The other agents do not affect exoerythrocytic forms of P. vivax.
6. _B_ Pyrimethamine acts by inhibiting dihydrofolate reductase (DHRI)
7. _D_ Chloroguanide (a DHRI) is metabolized to an active metabolite, chloroguanil.
8. _D_ Praziquantel is the drug of choice for intestinal cestode infestations.
9. _D_
10. _C_
11. _E_
12. _E_
13. _B_
14. _D_

CHAPTER 12: GASTROINTESTINAL DRUGS

1. _E_ The correct answer is castor oil. its acts generally within 2 hours and would cause distress. Methylcellulose, danthron, phenolphthalein and cascara are all long acting agents and one ingesting these substances could be expected to sleep through the night.

2. _D_ The correct answer would be either methyl or carboxymethylcellulose. These agents could swell as they pass through the esophagus, water helps flush them rapidly into the stomach.

3. _A_ The correct answer is mineral oil. Phenolphthalein can cause allergies and the magnesium salts cause side effects only in the presence of abnormal renal function.

4. _D_ Antacids indirectly decrease pepsin activity by increasing the pH of the stomach to above 4. Antacids are used for treatment of hyperchlorhydria and they are weak bases. Antacids with aluminum or calcium content also have a direct inhibitory effect on pepsin activity.

5. _B_ The correct answer is increased tone of the GI tract. Reduced tone is of therapeutic benefit when atropine-like compounds are used in ulcer therapy but side effects occur well before the high concentrations needed to affect acid secretion can be administered.

6. _A_ The correct answer is an opium alkaloid. Of the agents listed, opium is effective for treatment of severe diarrhea or dysentery. Opium acts to directly reduce the tone and motility of the GI tract. Kaolin, pectin and bismuth subcarbonate are adsorbents and have no direct action on the GI tract. They are generally less effective for severe diarrhea or dysentery.

7. _A_ Hydroxyzine and chlorpromazine are antiemetics. Diphenhydramine is an antihistamine and nabilone is a cannabinoid derivative used in cancer therapy.

8. _A_ Sodium bicarbonate is an absorbable antacid while the others are not, unless renal function is impaired.

9. _A_

10. _B_

11. _A_

12. _E_

CHAPTER 13: RESPIRATORY DRUGS

1. _C_ Most clinical drug assays measure total drug concentrations, while only the free concentration is the effective form of the drug. The therapeutic range of theophylline in the adult is 10-20 µg/ml with an average protein binding of 56% resulting in a free concentration of 4.4 to 8.8 µg/ml. In the infant theophylline protein binding is about 36%. The same free concentration of 4.4 to 8.8 µg/ml give a total plasma (free + bound) concentration of 6.6 to 11.0 µg/ml.

2. _D_

3. _B_ Pancrelipase is used in pancreatic deficiency in cystic fibrosis or chronic pancreatitis. Rifampin, which inhibits bacterial RNA synthesis, is used in treating tuberculosis.

4. _E_

5. _D_

6. _B_

7. _E_

8. _A_

9. _C_

CHAPTER 14: DRUGS ACTING ON THE UTERUS

1. _E_ Dihydroertgotamine
2. _C_ Caffeine
3. _D_ Methysergide
4. _E_ Ergotamine
5. _B_ Magnesium sulfate
6. _D_ Oxytocin
7. _E_ Ritodrine
8. _C_ Carboprost tromethamine
9. _A_ Methylergonovine

CHAPTER 15: TOXICOLOGY

1. _A_ Dimercaprol
2. _D_ Trientine
3. _C_ First trimester
4. _C_ Mercury
5. _E_ Deferoxamine
6. _I_ Penicillamine is one of two orally effective chelating agents for copper. The other in trientine.
7. _E_ Ethanol competes for alcohol dehydrogenase, the enzyme which initiates metabolism of methanol and glycols to toxic metabolites.

CHAPTER 15 (Continued)

8. _F_ Flumazenil is a specific benzodiazepine antagonist.
9. _B_ Apomorphine is given by s.c. injection for rapid emesis. Both emesis and CNS depression are blocked by naloxone
10. _N_ Succimer is indicated for lead poisoning in children. Penicillamine (choice I) is an alternative correct answer, but allergic reactions are fairly common.
11. _K_ Phytonadione is an injectable form of vitamin K_1.
12. _H_ Amyl nitrate is given by inhalation; sodium nitrite is given by i.v. infusion.
13. _J_ Physostigmine is the antidote for atropine and other belladonna alkaloids.
14. _A_ Activated charcoal is given to prevent absorption of many organic toxins from the GI tract. The dose is limited only by tolerance of the patient.
15. _G_ Ipecac is given only orally; apomorphine only by injection.
16. _M_ Digoxin-specific antibody fragments are available.
17. _L_ Pralidoxime is a cholinesterase regenerating agent, and is indicated in cases of poisoning with organophosphate cholinesterase inhibitors such as parathion.

CHAPTER 16: VITAMINS

1. _C_
2. _D_
3. _B_
4. _E_
5. _A_
6. _D_
7. _B_
8. _E_
9. _C_
10. _A_

CHAPTER 17: U.S. DRUG LAWS

1. _E_ Class X
2. _B_ Department of Justice
3. _A_ None
4. _B_ One teaspoonful contains about 5 ml. The prescription would require (5 ml/dose) X(4 doses/day) X 7 days = 140 ml.